The Cartesian Split

The Cartesian Split examines the phenomenon of Cartesian influence as a psychological complex in the Jungian tradition. It explores the full legacy of Cartesian rationality in its emphasis on abstract thinking and masculinisation of thought, often perceived in a negative light, despite the developments of modernity.

The book argues that the Cartesian creation of the Modern Age, as accompanied by a radical dualism, is better understood as a myth while acknowledging the psychological reality of the myth. The Cartesian myth is a collective dream, and the urgency of its rhetoric suggests that an important message is being left unheeded. This message may lead us to answers in the most unexpected place of all. The book brings forth the Cartesian myth in a new context and shows it to have potential meaning for us today.

The book will be of great interest for academics, researchers, and post-graduate students in the fields of analytical psychology, mental health, comparative mythology, and Jungian studies.

Brandon D. Short is a mechanical engineer with an interest in psychology. He holds a doctorate of depth psychology from Pacifica Graduate Institute. He lives in Portland, Oregon, USA.

Research in Analytical Psychology and Jungian Studies Series

Series Advisor: Andrew Samuels, Professor of Analytical Psychology, Essex University, UK.

The *Research in Analytical Psychology and Jungian Studies* series features research-focused volumes involving qualitative and quantitative research, historical/archival research, theoretical developments, heuristic research, grounded theory, narrative approaches, collaborative research, practitioner-led research, and self-study. The series also includes focused works by clinical practitioners, and provides new research informed explorations of the work of C. G Jung that will appeal to researchers, academics, and scholars alike.

Books in this series:

Jungian Metaphor in Modernist Literature
Exploring Individuation, Alchemy and Symbolism
Roula-Maria Dib

Symbolic Mental Representations in Arts and Mystical Experiences
Primordial Mental Activity and Archetypal Constellations
Giselle Manica

Jung's Technique of Active Imagination and Desoille's Directed Waking Dream Method
Bridging the Divide
Laner Cassar

The Cartesian Split
A Hidden Myth
Brandon D. Short

For more information about this series please visit: https://www.routledge.com/Research-in-Analytical-Psychology-and-Jungian-Studies/book-series/JUNGIANSTUDIES.

The Cartesian Split

A Hidden Myth

Brandon D. Short

Routledge
Taylor & Francis Group
LONDON AND NEW YORK

First published 2021
by Routledge
2 Park Square, Milton Park, Abingdon, Oxon OX14 4RN

and by Routledge
605 Third Avenue, New York, NY 10017

Routledge is an imprint of the Taylor & Francis Group, an informa business

British Library Cataloguing-in-Publication Data
A catalogue record for this book is available from the British Library

Library of Congress Cataloging-in-Publication Data
A catalog record has been requested for this book

ISBN: 978-0-367-24593-1 (hbk)
ISBN: 978-0-429-28335-2 (ebk)

Typeset in Sabon
by codeMantra

To Cassandra

Contents

Figures

Preface

The Western academy has a father complex. This complex is deep and tumultuous, rife with emotion and resentment, while also compulsive and irrational. For sure, the academy has a long and respectable tradition, venerated and sophisticated, featuring some of the best minds doing some of the best research. But in this one respect, it is like a child that is overly fixated on its father, too obsessed with escaping his long shadow. This father is none other than René Descartes, the 17th-century philosopher now known as the "father of modern philosophy." In a postmodern age, he is the icon of modernity most commonly rejected, oftentimes with glee.

The father complex itself is perhaps best known as one half of the Oedipus complex. This was given to us from another father, Sigmund Freud, the father of psychoanalysis. In Freud's writings, the Oedipus complex looms ominously, present to some degree in nearly every case study. Deep down, says Freud, we all harbor deep resentment and antipathy toward our fathers. This idea is perhaps not so well accepted anymore, but it does offer a useful perspective on our collective attitude toward Descartes. In nearly every academic field, it is common to find an urgent exhortation, in some form or another, for a complete emancipation from Cartesian influence. It is presumed that such influence is widespread, pernicious in its effects, and must be singled out and rejected before any further progress can be made. In other words, this collective child of the Academy feels compelled to kill its father.

Although this complex is multi-faceted, one particular aspect of it is surely the infamous doctrine of Cartesian dualism. Of all the Cartesian ideas to reject, this is the one that seems to be the most urgent. Why? Often, it is assumed that this idea is not just a present problem but marks an unusually tragic event in Western history. It is believed that in previous epochs, the mind, or one's own inner self, was considered to be harmonious and contiguous with all other levels of existence. However, it is said, Descartes drove a stake through the heart of this original wholeness and divided it into two. This was not just substance dualism but a *radical* dualism. Mind was now *separate* from body, subject was now *separate* from object, and inner was now *separate* from outer. The soul itself, once the most privileged mode of existence, suddenly found itself split off and separated from nearly everything else. Contemporary critiques go to great lengths to show that this division into two was invalid and illegitimate. The child must kill the father by healing the split.

Some readers may object to me referring to this behavior as a complex, on several levels. For one, the commonplace usage of the term is usually reserved for individuals and not groups. Another, perhaps larger, objection might be toward the overall sense of validity. Often, the word "complex" is invoked to discredit an opinion, to reduce its claim of objectivity. But surely, such a rejection of dualism is "objectively" true? After all, there is a long line of highly respected figures who have made this critique, as I will show. They cannot all be acting out of some kind of a psychological error. Or can they? I will address these concerns and others throughout the book. For now, it is enough to state that, in spite of all the excellent work by these figures, there is yet something else.

What is missing is a full recognition that these critiques, however well argued, are based on a gross mischaracterization of Descartes' original philosophical arguments. It is not so much a distortion, however, as an additional story, overlaid on top of the historical facts. It is a subliminal, compulsive story, running throughout many such critiques, and has seemingly taken on a life of its own. It is like an internet meme gone viral, such that it has completely transcended its humble origins. Others have noticed this problem, and critiqued it, but it seems to live on, unperturbed. It is in this respect that I consider it to be a complex.

However, I wish to emphasize that I have no intention of denigrating these critiques. On the contrary, I consider them all to be highly valuable, precisely *because* it is a complex. I am suggesting that this complex is not so much bad philosophy as misunderstood fantasy, a hidden myth, hiding in plain sight. I will contend that it contains within it, at least potentially, a meaningful message. To recognize this, uncover it, and understand it better is the aim of this book.

Notably, this book is a work in psychology, but I do not intend it to be limited to a psychological audience. It is intended for all academic fields that have claimed an intellectual tradition that has been somehow influenced by Descartes. This range is far beyond just philosophy, extending as far as art history and religious studies. For such a wide audience, I will limit the use of specialized terminology specific to psychology. Instead, I intend to liberally employ metaphor and an intentional personifying of the contents of the study. In other words, I will attempt to tell a story, with subjects as much as concepts.

So, imagine if you will, a person named "Ash" who has decided to go into therapy. Ash is having trouble at work and in relationships, specifically with authority figures. Whenever a problem is encountered, in any life situation, it always seems to revolve around some leader or historical founder. When asked for more detail, Ash consistently recalls events from early childhood, especially those involving Ash's father, Rand. At these moments of the conversation, emotions are raised, and Ash's face becomes contorted and bitter. The therapist recognizes at once a textbook father complex. Yet the situation is also quite delicate, and so the first task is, crucially, to listen.

In this book, Ash is the Western academy, Rand is Descartes, and I hope to be the therapist. So now, I invite Ash to lie back, relax, and please, "tell me about your Father."

Epigraph

I had this dream, a big dream...

I am walking down the streets of my old neighborhood, until I come to my childhood house. But it was different. In the front yard, there were these two large stone hands coming out of the ground, cold and pale, one on the left and one on the right. Then, the sky darkened, a terrible wind gathered, and I was afraid. A huge Captain Hook figure rose up slowly from behind the house. He let out a maniacal, evil laugh, and a thunderbolt came crashing down, splitting the house into two. I think my mother was still in there. I was terrified, and tried to close my eyes, but something held my gaze. Nothing happened for a very long time. Then, something rises from beneath the rubble, right in the middle. It is a unicorn, untouched and unharmed. It levitates and floats gently in the breeze, staring right at me the whole time. I feel a sense of peace, but I do not know what to do. Then, I woke up.

Chapter 1

Introduction

The allure of the error

I remember the day well. I was strolling the aisles of my favorite bookstore, a very large bookstore, but one that still has a small bookshop feel. Noteworthy books will often get hand-written notes from the staff, placed under the stacks, guiding the shopper with useful commentary. On this day, one such note really caught my eye. It was underneath a popular book on modern neuroscience, titled *Descartes' Error*, by Antonio Damasio. The book had merited the title of "Staff's Picks," a glowing recommendation. But beyond this, the reviewer felt compelled to spend a little extra time on the note, to add a somewhat comical drawing of Descartes, looking something like this:

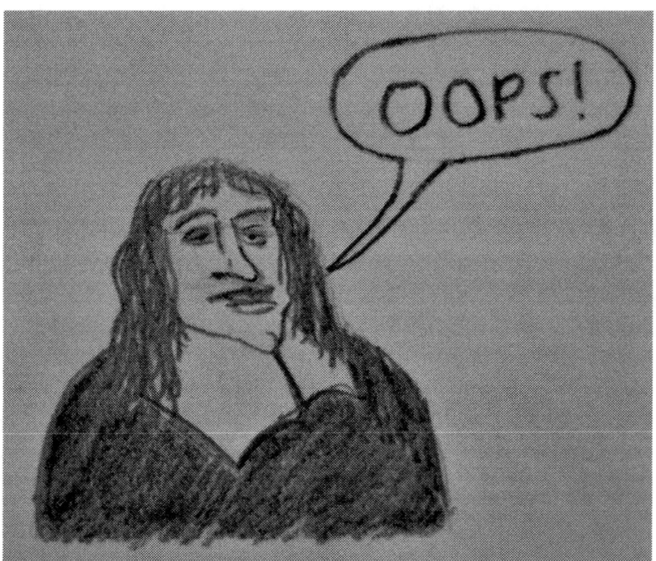

Figure 1.1 Author's impression of bookstore drawing.

At the time, the book was already a bestseller, but this hand-drawn image could have probably sold many more all by itself. The "OOPS!" says it all. How very tantalizing! Provocative! A relatively unknown neuroscientist had managed to expose the father of modern philosophy as fraudulent, foolish even. A legendary figure, required reading in every college philosophy class, was forced to humble himself before the miraculous discoveries of modern science, and sheepishly admit he got it all wrong.

Upon opening the book, in the very first pages, similar recommendations are found from professional reviewers. In particular, Damasio is celebrated for triumphantly overcoming the legendary influence of Cartesian thought. One reviewer states, "Damasio boldly challenges the dualisms that have dogged Western thought" (as cited in Damasio, 2006, p. i). In another edition, we learn that Damasio "cogently rejects simplistic divisions." The opportunity presented by this rejection is quite exciting. This "astonishing book. . . reveals the invisible world within us." It is a "revolutionary portrait," which "challenges the dogma." A call is issued to a wide range of scholars: "By all means, read this book" (as cited in Damasio, 1995, pp. i–iii).

The overall message is clear: Cartesian influence is widespread but is now recognized to be seriously flawed. While it may have helped contribute to modern science, with all of its accompanying benefits to humanity, now it is seen to be deeply harmful. Future progress depends on transcending this influence, to find a more holistic, natural, and reasonable conception of the human being. Who could possibly turn away from such a rich and promising proposition? It just *feels* like the right thing to do.

This basic feeling is at the core of my investigation. I have no interest in critiquing Damasio's neuroscientific findings, which are surely with merit. However, I do wish to investigate this feeling, the general tone of "anti-Cartesianism," that clearly accompanies the book, both on the cover and on the shelf.

It is fair to ask why a feeling, especially one with such broad acceptance, should become a research subject in its own right. One reason is that, for all its supposed importance, it is surprisingly ephemeral, and difficult to locate precisely. For example, upon opening the book, there is a conspicuous lack of anything related to Descartes. The infamous philosopher does not even show up until the final five pages. Even Damasio (1995) himself acknowledges that the formative stuff of the book "was neither about Descartes nor about philosophy" (p. xix). But for some reason, he felt compelled to name it after him and his egregious error. Why? I suspect it is for the same reason that the bookstore artist felt compelled to draw an amusing caricature of the intended target.

Whether Damasio was aware of it or not, this general tone of anti-Cartesianism is very popular, and naming the book along these lines probably helped to secure a warm reception to the book, and among a very broad audience. For one particular example of this, the book has been enthusiastically endorsed by Daniel Dennett (1995), a philosopher of mind and a prominent voice in modern consciousness studies. Dennett's own view is heavily materialistic, famously stating that consciousness is an illusion, and this is quite harmonious with Damasio's rejection of Descartes' *cogito*. Meanwhile, in a corner of the academy very far removed from Dennett, there is Coppin and Nelson's (2005) *The Art of Inquiry*. This small book, focused on qualitative research methodology, also advocates for Damasio, although for a very different reason. Coppin and Nelson are concerned that qualitative research has become too dry and technical, emulating the hard sciences too much, and as such, has lost its soul. Damasio's book is celebrated, because it confirms a holistic conception of the human psyche, "the bodymind," where soul is not separate from body (pp. 154–155). With this view, qualitative research can become more like the arts, more aesthetic and romantic, welcoming the soul back in.

I should not have to state that the audiences of these two books are quite different. Among the audience of the latter book, Dennett's rigorous materialism is usually met with a certain hostility. On the other hand, Dennett would probably not be too moved by the critique that anything scientific has lost its soul. Although there are surely some things in Damasio's book that are agreeable to both audiences, I suspect that the title of the book has significantly increased the chances of a positive evaluation, regardless of the audience and their background. In this case, as it is often the case with Descartes, the enemy of my enemy is my (unacknowledged) friend.

This feeling of anti-Cartesianism is broad, extending into many other fields, and interestingly, it has remarkable staying power. Damasio's "revolutionary" book came out in 1994, became a best-seller, and gained broad approval. It has also reached far beyond academic confines; you can even buy t-shirts online featuring the book's title ("Descartes Error—Mixed Mental Arts—T-Shirt | TeePublic," 2019). Once an idea has reached this kind of mass penetration, it would seem safe to say that the victory has been won. Ostensibly, Cartesian influence should have been eliminated by now, or at least, clearly sequestered.

And yet, the revolution goes on; 24 years after Damasio's book was published, an article appeared in the online *Psychology Today,* which seems to call for a similar pointed rejection, all over again. In this article, McCann and Bechsgaard (2018) generally recapitulate the overall feeling of Damasio's book, or at least the front cover, as I have summarized above. They call for a wholesale rejection of Cartesian influence, almost as if Damasio's book was never written. The article ends with a nice summation, and a poignant image, and so is worth restating it in whole:

> The call for the rejection of this limited view is coming from a variety of quarters.... We urgently need to replace the machine metaphor which has re-shaped how we see both the human body and the human mind.

> We need to break up with Rene Descartes. The letter might go something like this:
>
> Dear Rene,
>
> It has been an eventful 500 years and we have been through a lot together. As exhilarating as it has been it is time for us to go our separate ways.
>
> Sincerely, the Western World (para. 7)

And yet, given the ongoing nature of this rejection, it is perhaps easier said than done. Perhaps we have solemnly realized that we are in an abusive relationship, but we are too far in it to be willing to undergo a difficult break-up. According to a book titled *Goodbye, Descartes*, we learn that Cartesian influence is so deeply "ingrained in the psyche of twentieth-century Western man that any theory that challenges that view is bound to have a hard time of it" (Devlin, 1998, p. 279). This, of course, does not dissuade Devlin, and others, from valiantly trying. Perhaps all of these authors are simply doing what they can, chipping away at the old harmful edifice, one brick at a time, taking the long view of faith that one fine day will bring the final emancipation. Regardless, it seems the feeling of anti-Cartesianism can draw a powerful, long-lasting interest.

The split in the middle

The scope of my investigation must be focused further. Simply "anti-Cartesianism," in all its varied forms, is much too broad. For whatever reason, Descartes has always been an unusually big target, from times long before Damasio. He has been "attacked, reviled, and condemned like no other thinker for most of the last 350 years" (Bracken, 2002, p. 1). To make things more difficult, he has also been a moving target. Gaukroger (1998) states, "more than any other modern philosopher, he has been fashioned according to the philosophies of the time and interpreted accordingly" (p. 3). For example, Descartes drew the ire of many of his contemporaries, including both Voltaire and Pascal, but for different reasons from each other, and for very different reasons than we have today. Even if I were to restrict my study to only current sources, I could not possibly account for all the unusually harsh critiques levied at Descartes.

However, there is one modern critique in particular that can be defined and recognized precisely. It is the usual argument against Cartesian dualism, but with much more colorful rhetoric, and strikingly more dramatic claims. It is in fact no longer an argument, but a vehement rejection; no longer a debate in philosophy, but an existential crisis. It is the urgent call to transcend the radical Cartesian *Split*.

This new target is perhaps exemplified by Walker Percy (1999), in his novel *Love in the Ruins*. In it, the protagonist feels he has finally realized the solution to this age-old problem, as he scribbles feverishly in his notebook:

> Hear the triumphant news. . . the first hope of bridging the dread chasm that has rent the soul of Western man ever since the famous philosopher Descartes ripped body loose from mind and turned the very soul into a ghost that haunts its own house.
>
> (p. 191)

As I will show later, there are many variants of this notion, but this image of disastrous and tragic separation, or specifically, a "split," can be seen as a convenient common thread. Perhaps all the other critiques are related to this, but the split serves as a highly useful focal point. For example, Damasio (1995) himself nicely echoes this sentiment when he finally defines Descartes' error as "the *abyssal* separation between body and mind" [italics added] (p. 249). And so, there is a widespread and urgent interest in overcoming Cartesian influence, and now there is a specific target of that rejection, the legendary Cartesian Split. The split must be transcended, or healed, if we are to go on. Ironically, if we were to go through with the break-up with Descartes, this would amount to healing the split by splitting up.

This irony should give us pause. Before we split up with Descartes, we should first understand what exactly he split up. There are many ways to approach this, but perhaps it is best, again, to begin with the focal point, these images of dread chasms and abysses. To put it simply, such images have very little to do with actual Cartesian philosophy. In spite of these author's good scholarship in other areas, the idea that Descartes argued for such a profound and radical separation, is just that, an idea. This interpretation, if it can be called that, is drastically out of step with most of the dedicated commentary on the subject.

Among philosophers, for example, there is widespread agreement that Descartes argued for a *distinction* between mind and body, rather than a *separation*. There is also wide agreement that, in addition to this distinction, he also argued for a rather intimate, two-way causal interaction between body and mind. The usual critique in this community is not so much against dualism *per se*, but that Descartes failed to convince on the manner of the interaction, or made some fatal logical error, such as the Cartesian circle. Third, the common interpretation of Descartes' "mind," the *cogito*, is quite different than in most of the above sources. For Damasio, for example, *cogito* means abstract, intellectual thinking, or the kind of thinking opposed to the emotions. Whereas, for most philosophers, *cogito* includes the emotions.

While even this interpretation is problematic, which I will address later, it is important to note at this point that the notion of a radical split, is simply not found in the source texts. On the contrary, in the 6th meditation, Descartes (1984) details how the mind and body are united.

To illustrate this, he uses a metaphor of a sailor on a ship, representing mind on a body. This is perhaps a metaphor that could be used by many today. In this metaphor, the mind and body are connected, but it turns out that the manner of connection does not suit Descartes. Interestingly, he argues for an even more intimate union than this would allow. He states, "I am not merely present in my body as a sailor is present in a ship, but that I am very closely joined and, as it were, intermingled with it, so that I and the body form a unit" (p. 56). Further, the activity of such an "I" implies more than just the intellect. Descartes defines "thinking" as the activity of that which "doubts, understands, affirms, denies, is willing, is unwilling, and also imagines and has sensory perceptions" (p. 19).

So, is all this misunderstanding simply poor scholarship on behalf of those like Damasio? I do not think this is the appropriate judgment. Such a judgment might be sound if it was an isolated instance, but in one form or another, this kind of "poor scholarship" seems to prevail much too mightily. It occurs too frequently, and among too many distinguished academics. While others have recognized this problem, it is usually given little attention, or attributed to "nothing but" poor scholarship. I believe that the overall phenomenon deserves to be a research topic all on its own and that some other explanation for it is required. My basic point of departure is this: Regardless of the truth of these claims, *people seem to want it to be true*. It is this general desire that is perhaps fueling Damasio's raucous approval. It is the allure of finding and following a new, brave pioneer, one who has managed to bridge a 400-year-old unbridgeable chasm. This feeling, this desire, is the entry point to the Cartesian Split complex, and this needs its own framing, understanding, and interpretation.

Approaching the split

At this point, my imaginary consulting room may be invoked again, to help clarify my unique approach to this issue. The therapist believes Ash has a father complex, and fittingly, most of the stories Ash tells of Rand are simply incredulous. Ash tells stories of Rand's extreme violence, in some cases, of an almost inhuman nature. Ash also believes that Rand is responsible for pitting one half of the family against the other, such that neither side ever interacts with the other anymore. Rand is told to be very powerful, having influenced every decision made in the entire city. This is also very curious, for, according to Ash, he was also quite idiotic, easily confused, and unable to win any argument with anyone.

The therapist knows enough about human nature to know that no one human could possibly amount to that much terrible influence. Patients in therapy are often known to exaggerate their memories and personal stories. But the therapist is also skilled enough to know that it is not helpful at all to simply say, "oh come now, surely your father is not so bad. You are simply exaggerating, imagining it, and projecting your own problems onto the memories of your real father. The real problem is not with him, *but with you.*"

No, such a cold and unsympathetic statement would drive Ash straight out of the consulting room and onto the next personal disaster. The statement may be essentially true, but the therapist also knows that, in spite of all these unbelievable claims, the stories *feel real enough to Ash at the time.* In other words, it is probably not true that Rand did those things, but, regardless, *it is true* that Ash remembers things that way, and so the therapist has to play along for a bit. Perhaps there is a dark part of Ash's psyche, something long forgotten and repressed, but at the same time, important for Ash's future development. Perhaps such a thing is demanding attention to itself by creating a false story out of Rand memories, disclosing itself as real by precisely not being real. The therapist must not belittle the fantasy, but rather, see where it leads.

It is the same way with our collective fantasy about Descartes. I believe in order to fully unpack the Cartesian Split complex, you have to be incredulous and trusting at the same time. In other words, it is not true that Descartes made an "abyssal separation." And yet, it is true that people uncritically believe it. In order to understand the true meaning, you have to temporarily accept this false belief. This is a very subtle position to take, and I hope this therapeutic example can be continuously recalled, in order to keep this position in mind.

Earlier, I framed this subject through the lens of Freud, via the father complex. However, I should be more clear about the full range of my influences, and my own usage of them for this study. It is better to say that my approach is not so much psychoanalytical but depth psychological. With this term, I am incorporating not just Freud but also Carl Gustav Jung, the Swiss psychologist who followed Freud. Despite their differences, both theorists employ an overall conception of the human psyche in which various unconscious forces operate independently of the conscious process, and can interfere with it, in problematic ways. This is manifested in various irrational behaviors, which can operate at both the individual and cultural levels. Such behavior is characterized by distorted perceptions of reality and preferred versions of history, even if recognized to be harmful or incomplete. Further, such behavior is unusually persistent, even after having been challenged by others. It is in these common respects that the problematic cultural interpretation of Descartes can be fruitfully understood.

My specific approach, however, is more informed by Jung than Freud. Jung distinguished his approach from Freud by minimizing the focus on frustrated biological drives, occurring only in early childhood. Although he agreed on the importance of such activity, he ultimately regarded it as a secondary influence. For Jung, the unconscious is not created from frustrated adolescence, but is pre-existing, and can also act constructively for further development. As part of this new model, Jung emphasized his notion of archetypes and the collective unconscious. Jung conceived of archetypes as innate structuring principles, operating at the deepest level of the psyche, and common to all humanity. They are also closely connected to the expression of human instincts. It is from this deeper, more powerful layer of the psyche, that gives the complex its power.

My approach is also influenced by James Hillman, the American psychologist who was active in the late 20th century. Hillman began his career in the Jungian school, but later played a prominent role in forming a distinct branch, named archetypal psychology. One of the distinguishing features of this approach is an increased level of attention toward the precise details of the psychological phenomenon under study. The keyword for this focus is *image*. Hillman (1992) warns that abstract, technical interpretations tend to become literalized and dogmatic, which can obscure important information contained in the original image (pp. 144–145).

This particular approach may be best demonstrated by example. Perhaps Ash comes to the first therapy session after having a big dream the night before. In this dream, Ash was in front of a house from the distant past, but recognizable, perhaps from childhood. Ash then looks up at the house in terror, seeing a huge, distorted image of Rand, who splits the house right down the middle. Ash's mother is feared to be inside.

In the initial session, Ash is understandably distraught recounting the details of this terrible dream. It would be a grave mistake for the therapist to say, "the splitting is merely your own father complex, reflecting your own internal dissociation." Rather, the archetypal psychologist would gently say, "tell me more about Rand's face," or, "what does the house look like now?" With this approach, the specific choices of words used by the dreamer are focused on, and not so hastily bypassed for theory. The words are understood as being pregnant with potential meaning, and studied closely. I intend to follow this approach in this book.

The approach of archetypal psychology also implies a different scope for what typically comes under the term "therapy." Hillman was trained as a personal therapist, but later was more interested in the "therapy of ideas," and his later writings reflect this. This approach would seem natural, for if archetypes are innate and universal, then they are necessarily active in all human activity, and not just in the moments of psychotherapy. In other words, anything involving human thinking is open to archetypal influence. Interestingly, this approach is contained in Jung, but not the Jung that most people are familiar with. Shamdasani (2003) argues that Jung himself intended for his ideas to be applied outside of personal therapy. Indeed, it appears he even hoped for founding of a general psychology that could be applied to any discipline whatsoever. He even appeared to have chosen a unique term for it, that of "complex psychology," within which personal therapy is only one part (pp. 13–15). From this perspective, a widespread cultural phenomenon of mistaken philosophical interpretation can indeed be seen as a collective activity of complexes, and also approached with a methodology particular to complexes.

The complexity of complexes

It may prove to be regrettable that Jung's offered moniker was not chosen, for there is a wealth of insight available within the term "complex." The full range of potential meanings, and their implications, is itself, well, complex. For one, the term can be taken as value-neutral, especially in Jung's formulation. Contrary to popular understanding, having a complex does not necessarily imply that something has gone wrong. In Jung's usage of the term, complexes are the basic structural units of the psyche, inherent to all its processes. Indeed, the ego is itself a complex. "A complex becomes pathological only when we think we have not got it" (Jung, 1943/1985, p. 79).

A complex can also be regarded positively, as an expression of undeveloped potential. For example, it may very well be that Rand was a bad father, but perhaps Ash's other siblings do not feel the need to blame everything on him. Perhaps in Ash's unique personal life, there is a need for some reason to develop more authoritative skills, and the potential to do so has formed a father complex around the figure of Rand, in Ash's own imagination. The complex can then be seen as a positive development, a sign that further maturation is on the way, and the pathological behavior is simply a way to ensure appropriate attention is given to the development of these latent skills.

Complexes also tend to be bipolar, able to hold a pair of conflicting ideas somehow in unison. Recall that Ash believed Rand to be almost superhumanly powerful, holding entire communities under his influence. But at the same time, Ash refers to Rand as being foolish, illogical, and incompetent, at even the most basic tasks. One wonders how such a person could actually exist, but it seems to have no problem existing in Ash's psyche. This kind of behavior alone hints at a range of unexplored meanings and potential behind the image.

Complexes tend to magnify otherwise small events into something much larger, becoming blown all out of proportion. Perhaps Ash painfully recalls a particular memory of Rand as a bad father, perhaps losing his patience one day and throwing away Ash's favorite toy. Now this event may turn out to be historically true, but most parents have regrettable moments such as this. The curious question is then: Why should Ash feel so traumatized, today, by such a commonplace event, that happened so many years ago?

Although complexes can reflect a true event, it is usually the departure from historical reality that offers the most amount of insight. Complexes often exaggerate and distort the facts to such a degree that the link to the original historical event can be very difficult to comprehend. It is more likely that Rand took away a small plastic toy for one day, because Ash was simply misbehaving. But perhaps the story has mutated over the years into something much more malevolent, such as Rand burning Ash's most treasured possession, and having Ash watch him do it, laughing the whole time, while Ash cried. Suddenly, an otherwise normal human being in the past has become a supervillain, something more likely to be found in a fairy tale featuring an evil sorcerer.

Another curious aspect of such a story might be Ash's insistence on its historical truth. Perhaps Ash would insist on the memory being exactly as it happened, expressing no doubts, especially when doubt in this case would be very reasonable. Most adults cannot remember events perfectly from only the prior month, much less from early childhood. But in this case, Ash may insist loudly that the events transpired exactly as recalled in memory, and any attempt to cast doubt on the veracity of the story is met with scorn and derision. Ash has suddenly become a memory expert, even if not otherwise justified, and to this we can all relate.

Complexes are not only personal but can extend easily into the collective sphere. This should seem natural, as a collection of individuals is also a collection of individual psyches, and collective events such as discussions and arguments are also psychic events. But for whatever reason, even within many Jungian scholars, complexes tend to be understood and discussed at only the personal level. This is probably related to the fact that Jungian thought has been more prolific at the therapeutic level instead of at the general academic. However, in recent years, several Jungian scholars have been exploring the notion of "cultural complexes," most prominently Singer and Kimbles, who also coined the term (Kirsch, 2004, p. 185). Although the range of application of these complexes is obviously different, the overall dynamic is remarkably similar to personal complexes, and most of the prior examples I have given with Ash also apply to groups. This is of course fitting, as I introduced the figure of Ash explicitly as a representative of Western academia.

Complexes also tend to be somewhat difficult to work with, requiring alternate modes of engagement. Often, if a complex is approached within its original frames of reference, various defense mechanisms may be activated, which prevent any real productive developments. This is one reason why dreams and other activities of the imagination are valuable in therapy. Such expressions can provide an alternate outlet for the underlying issue, such that old problems may be confronted in a new way. This is another reason for working with the Ash metaphor.

Finally, complexes tend to thrive in places where you least expect to find them. Psychotherapists themselves are certainly not immune to them. Kirsch (2004) understands the bitter 100-year feud between the Jungian and Freudian communities as a cultural complex itself. Of course, this feud resulted from a past trauma, the conveniently titled "split," between these two great thinkers. Also, Hillman (1978), in his *Myth of Analysis*, marked out early territory for his archetypal psychology by arguing that psychotherapy itself was suffering, and in need of therapy. In other words, the very language that was supposed to be able to decipher unconscious content was itself pregnant with unconscious meaning. Only, perhaps to prove his point, Hillman did not even trust the term "unconscious." If professional psychologists are unaware of their own hidden stories, even existing within their very own language, then certainly philosophers can be too.

In summary, complexes, in the Jungian sense, are certainly more than what they seem. One never has "just a father complex," but instead is invoking with those words a very wide range of potential understanding. Complexes are both pathological and promising, both true and fanciful. They can hold conflicting ideas within a single reference, and can do so both personally and collectively, and are omnipresent. All such dynamics are at play with the Cartesian Split complex, and the examples provided with Ash and Rand were written specifically to bring these dynamics to life. The connections between the Cartesian Split complex and the metaphorical story will be drawn out in more detail throughout the book. The reader may benefit from reviewing the examples above after having completed the exposition in the book.

Cogito ergo non sum

My own history with this subject extends long before my stroll through the bookstore. As an early student, I was thoroughly enamored with math and science, and for me, Descartes was a hero. I loved the precision of mathematics, and for quite some time, I was of the opinion that truth was only to be found in exact calculations. In English class, we might have read a poem, and spent the rest of the day speculating on what the author meant. Although this was interesting, I was troubled by the thought that all such opinions were inherently untrustworthy. How can anyone, including my teacher, claim to have the "right" interpretation? Could such an interpretation ever be proved to be right? And if so, what were the criteria? Worse, if it turned out that there was no such thing as a right interpretation, how were we all not just wasting our time?

By contrast, there was no such doubt with math. Two plus three was five, exactly five, and that was the right answer. This process, for me, was the epitome of elegance. I also remember well the first time I learned the Cartesian coordinate system, and how you could use it to model the behavior of natural motion. I remember going outside and throwing objects in the air, and with only a stopwatch, I could calculate how high it went, as well as the speed at which it left my hand. I could do all this with one simple equation. The realization that I could understand such a relationship, between calculations and measurement, was thrilling to me. This fascination was present in me as a small child and extended through most of my adult life. I graduated from college with a degree in mechanical engineering, and have been employed as an engineer ever since.

On the other hand, throughout my early life, I sometimes displayed tendencies that were opposed to these rational ideals. Throughout engineering school, I harbored a doubt that even the mathematical process, however powerful, did not lead to the ultimate truth. On the contrary, I suspected that math and science may actually inhibit the search for it. I suspected that the really big questions of life, including even the meaning of life, were far beyond what could be calculated. Out of sight from my engineering peers, I secretly read books on religion and philosophy. I even flirted with Eastern mysticism, which emphasized the profound truth of "not-knowing." One of my favorite engineering classes was on the philosophy of science, in which we briefly touched upon the parable of Plato's cave, and that the mind was more real than things. This was a profound realization for me. What if, all of those previous moments of certainty were nothing but shadows dancing on the wall?

In spite of those doubts on the side, my identity as an engineer was firmly in place, until a period of time in my early thirties. I ended up in a very dark place. Many of my life goals, that of relationships, career, and hobbies, had all ended in failure. Worse, I felt trapped in these failures, and I fell into a deep depression. I questioned many things, but in particular, I became deeply disenchanted toward my chosen career path. I believed that an exclusive emphasis on rationality had led me to a fractured state of being, where I had lost something vitally important. Worse, I felt traumatized by it, feeling as if I had little to no access to the richer, deeper aspects of personhood, such as the arts. I read more and more books on alternative subjects, and many of these identified Descartes as the singular fountainhead of a Western paradigm that had led us all astray. I fell into this narrative. One particular morning, I felt particularly incensed toward this figure of Descartes, who surely had influenced the whole of Western culture, and therefore, the whole trajectory of my life. I believed on that day that Cartesian philosophy had a fundamental flaw in it, which has troubled us, and me, ever since. The essence of the human could not possibly be thinking. Rather, the opposite must be true; the mystics and artists had it right. I scribbled in my notebook my mantra for the week: *Cogito ergo non sum.*

Fortunately, I was able to make it out of that depression, and I now have a much more nuanced opinion of my interests and life choices. Although continuing as an engineer, I was able to make space for the so-called "non-rational" inclinations of my being. I was very excited when I first stumbled upon Jung, for this was a discipline that appeared to offer a path for both of my interests. Jung claimed emphatically that he was a scientist, doing empirical research, but incredibly, his research topics were dreams and myths! I was completely enthralled. Within a year, I charted out a course to go to graduate school and study depth psychology, without any concrete vocational goals. The experience was highly educational, but also, very healing. I felt I had finally found a path that could unify two seemingly disparate parts of my personality.

It did not take long during my new coursework to encounter once again a familiar face to me, the nefarious villain Descartes. Depth psychology is considered by many to have a strong kinship to postmodernism, and most postmodern inventories into the past locate Descartes' work as a singularly tragic turn. Although I was clearly sympathetic to the overall postmodern, psychological movement, I now felt some strong reservations to this specific account. Even though I had that original mantra moment, I felt that I had since embraced a larger perspective. From this new stance, I could now sense that there was a *disproportionate* amount of criticism and bitterness directed toward Descartes, over and above all the other "modern" sources. This time, I was able to remember my childhood Descartes, who was not a villain, but a hero, *in addition* to my mantra of the week. Although I was never trained in actual Cartesian philosophy, I began to doubt Descartes could be the source of so much gone wrong. But at the same time, I fully appreciated the need for a "post-Cartesian" worldview.

After several years of pondering this, I allowed myself to ask a simple question: Was Descartes really a Cartesian? This question felt dangerous and heretical to me at the time. I felt that doubting this assertion was placing me in singular opposition against the entire Western academy. I tentatively and hesitantly did research on this question, entering it exactly as phrased above, into an internet search engine. I did not really know what I was looking for. But what I found changed everything, and led me down the path to writing this book.

A complex offering

And now, dear reader, I trust you know enough about me and my story, but I do not know enough about you. Perhaps you have also raised doubts on this popular but questionable narrative? Or perhaps you are still doubting my hypothesis? After all, as I can attest, questioning one of the Western academy's most foundational narratives is a lot to ask.

But perhaps you also know enough about psychology yourself to suspect that this is nothing but my own personal complex, being projected onto the topic. I intentionally included all the messy details of my personal story, even though they might specifically invite such a suspicion. I fully admit to having a complex, it did require therapy, and it clearly revolved around "Cartesian" topics. Although I cannot claim to be fully healed from my complex, I do feel that my experiences with the subject allow me to have a unique, more nuanced perspective on the matter, perhaps one that is needed. But what is this need? What can my own psychological musings, spurred on from my own personal difficulties and haphazard web searches, contribute to centuries of philosophical criticism on one of the most widely read figures of the modern era?

Essentially, what I found on that one particular web search was that I was certainly not alone. Regardless of how they came to it, I found several others who have also come to the same suspicion. Somehow, somewhere along the line, a gross mischaracterization of Descartes was generated in the academy, then accepted in the academy, and has persisted ever since. I also learned that the problem is not limited to those outside of philosophy. There are several prominent voices in academic philosophy who, according to their colleagues, have constructed and solidified a partial and highly problematic interpretation of the original writings.

Perhaps the most prominent of these arguments is *Descartes' Dualism*, written by Gordon Baker and Katherine Morris (2002), professors of philosophy at Oxford. This book, along with others, is what I found on my tentative internet search. Although I will expand on this work and others like it in later sections, it is worth now summarizing some of their most salient observations. Simply stated, they answered my question in the negative. "Close textual analysis does not directly support. . . that Descartes held the main tenets of so-called 'Cartesian Dualism.'" Additionally, they suggest that a quasi-psychological force, a phenomenon they refer to as "the Cartesian Legend," seems to be acting somewhat autonomously, perpetuating this false interpretation (pp. 1–2). Incredibly, they found that many of the quotes often used to support this interpretation often contain within them elements that contradict it (p. 23). The "real" Descartes, if such a thing can even be conceived, may actually be farther away than ever.

At the same time, from a psychological perspective, the "unreal" Descartes is as real as ever. If there is a consistently flawed interpretation, with persistence and irony, even among the professionals, then there is very likely to be some kind of psychological mechanism involved. I will eventually leave it up to the philosophers to discover the "real" Descartes, but before such an effort can be made, I consider it fruitful to understand all possible mechanisms that have precluded the discovery in the first place. Baker and Morris's book is a work in philosophy, but the "Legend" clearly invites a psychological lens, particularly a depth psychological lens. Although they do a masterful job of describing the phenomenon from within their own framework, they are necessarily limited in fully exploring it, on its own terms. Essentially, this book is an attempt to do just that, and this is my hopeful contribution toward the ongoing discussion. My own complex has led me to such an investigation. Whatever has led you to me, let us now investigate together.

Outline of chapters

In the second and third chapters, I present the most prominent source material of the Cartesian Split cultural complex. This consists of all the various distortions, inaccuracies, and problematic interpretations. Thus far, I have provided brief justifications as to why such material can be considered as a complex. This overall justification will be further developed throughout the book, but the primary goal of these chapters is to simply document the material, at face value. In other words, it is best at this time to simply inventory and summarize the prominent commentary on the subject, regardless of whether or not the claims are factually true. This is the listening stage of the therapy. Occasionally, however, I will present some challenges to the claims, in order to demonstrate how it is part of a complex. Hopefully, throughout these chapters, the complex will progressively resemble more of a myth, something being uncovered from underneath the claims.

The fourth chapter summarizes the commentary of those who have recognized the overall misunderstanding but have left certain gaps in developing it. These sources are mostly from dedicated scholars of philosophy. Generally, past commentators either do not see it as much of problem, or do not fully appreciate the psychological nuances, and this is what I hope to supplement. I will also show that the matter is gaining attention, and as part of this, some have even employed a certain psychological approach, if without all the professional accoutrements, and without the necessary next steps. The remaining gaps and connections will be filled in as needed, in order to set up the remaining work.

In the fifth chapter, I delve into comparable activities of our collective imagination, specifically that of myth, in order to gain perspective on this new cultural product, the Cartesian myth. The human mind, for all its complexities, often demonstrates remarkable similarities, or patterns, in its various products. This can be shown to be the case between cultures separated from each other, in both time and space. Naturally, this draws heavily on archetypal theory, which I will also introduce in more detail, before such an inventory. I also analyze the Cartesian myth in terms of its essential features and present it as a composite of two different mythical strands.

The sixth chapter is the most psychological, in which I investigate the core meaning of the Cartesian Split cultural complex. In other words, the mythic strands are translated and interpreted into modern-day psychological terminology, specifically psychodynamic terminology used by Freud and Jung. While this move may be controversial, or perhaps somewhat arcane to outside audiences, I will demonstrate how it nonetheless offers a necessary additional perspective.

The seventh chapter attempts to locate the particular instance of this complex against a particular cultural context. It will be shown that the complex is more restrictive than is commonly assumed, and that these restrictions can be focused on in order to understand the subject more fully. In the process, however, various cultural and historical complexities are introduced, which perhaps complicate the study. As such, this chapter is highly speculative but suffices as at least a starting point for further investigation.

The eighth and final chapter serves two purposes. The first is to review and summarize the primary material and conclusions drawn throughout the book. The second is to revisit the original subject matter, the original words put on paper, concerning the now infamous substance dualism. My hope is that through the process of re-evaluation, a new perspective on an old topic yields fresh insight, perhaps toward our relevant needs today.

References

Baker, G. P., & Morris, K. J. (2002). *Descartes' dualism.* London, UK: Routledge.

Bracken, H. M. (2002). *Descartes.* Oxford, UK: Oneworld.

Coppin, J., & Nelson, E. (2005). *The art of inquiry: A depth psychological perspective* (2nd ed.). Putnam, CT: Spring Publication.

Damasio, A. R. (1995). *Descartes error: Emotion, reason and the human brain.* New York, NY: Avon Books.

Damasio, A. R. (2006). *Descartes error: Emotion, reason and the human brain.* London, UK: Vintage Books.

Dennett, D. (1995). Review of Damasio, Descartes' error. In *Times literary supplement* (pp. 3–4). Retrieved from: https://ase.tufts.edu/cogstud/dennett/papers/damasio.htm

Descartes Error—Mixed Mental Arts—T-Shirt | TeePublic. (2019, November 6). Retrieved November 6, 2019, from TeePublic website: https://www.teepublic.com/t-shirt/1232748-descartes-error

Descartes, R. (1984). *The philosophical writings of Descartes* (Vol. 2; J. Cottingham, R. Stoothoff, & D. Murdoch, Trans.). Cambridge, UK: Cambridge University Press.

Devlin, K. (1998). *Goodbye, Descartes: The end of logic and the search for a new cosmology of the mind.* New York, NY: Wiley.

Gaukroger, S. (1998). *Descartes: An intellectual biography.* Oxford, UK: Clarendon Press.

Hillman, J. (1978). *The myth of analysis: Three essays in archetypal psychology.* New York, NY: Harper Colophon.

Hillman, J. (1992). *Re-visioning psychology.* New York, NY: Harper Perennial.

Jung, C. G. (1985). Psychotherapy and a philosophy of life. In R. F. C. Hull (Trans.), *The collected works of C. G. Jung* (Vol. 16, pp. 76–83). Princeton, NJ: Princeton University Press. (Original work published 1943)

Kirsch, T. (2004). Cultural complexes in the history of Jung, Freud and their followers. In T. Singer & S. L. Kimbles (Eds.), *The cultural complex: Contemporary Jungian perspectives on psyche and society* (pp. 185–195). London, UK: Routledge.

McCann, G., & Bechsgaard, G. (2018, September 30). It's time to break up with Descartes. Retrieved February 10, 2019, from Psychology Today website: https://www.psychologytoday.com/blog/return-stillness/201809/its-time-break-descartes

Percy, W. (1999). *Love in the ruins: The adventures of a bad Catholic at a time near the end of the world.* New York, NY: Picador.

Shamdasani, S. (2003). *Jung and the making of modern psychology: The dream of a science.* Cambridge, UK: Cambridge University Press.

Chapter 2

The initial sessions

The Cartesian Split is both everywhere and nowhere at the same time. By "everywhere," I am referring to the observation that it can be found in virtually every academic field, being implicated in a wide variety of unfortunate modern developments. At the time of this writing, a web search for the exact phrase "Cartesian split" yields over 18,000 results, and this obviously only reflects digital sources. Thus, it is clearly impossible to document every such instance. At best, I can only provide in this work a sample of what was most prominently available to me at the time. However, this should suffice, in order to establish a sense of the basic psychological dynamic at work.

In order to help focus my survey, I originally searched for only works with the phrase "Cartesian split" explicitly in the abstract or in the title. At the time, using a popular academic works search engine, I found 34 different works that met that specific criteria. These works came from many different disciplines, spanning the fields of anthropology, education, literature, art, history, medicine, sociology, law, public administration, environmental studies, psychology and psychotherapy. All such instances that I found described it in a particularly negative manner. Also, the fact that the phrase appears in the abstract or title demonstrates the importance that the authors have assigned to it.

The phrase was also used quite casually, without any qualifying conditions or definitions. This demonstrates that the authors assume that the phrase has a clearly and commonly understood meaning. As I will show, this assumption is wrong. I will demonstrate from this survey that the phrase has a very wide range of semiotic associations. It is so wide, in fact, *that I consider the phrase "Cartesian Split" to be practically meaningless.*

This suggestion is not novel. Even within the rigorous debates of philosophical dualism, Lokhorst (2016) states that Descartes' theory of the mind-body relationship was never clearly articulated, even in his own writings. Further, there are at least 12 different interpretations that have appeared in the secondary literature in philosophy. Depending on whom you read, Descartes' dualism is either hylomorphist, Platonist, trialistic, interactionist, parallelist, nonparallelist, occasionalist, epiphenomenalist, supervenientist, dual-aspect identity theory, idealist, or materialist. As Lokhorst explains:

> Each of these interpretations agrees with at least some passages in Descartes' writings, but none agrees with all of them. Taken together, they suggest that Descartes' philosophy of mind contains echoes of all theories that had been proposed before him and anticipations of all theories that were developed afterwards: it is a multi-faceted diamond in which all mind-body theories that have ever been proposed are reflected.
>
> (para. 36–38)

Such a multivalence of interpretation is magnified even further outside of philosophy, and especially so when the word "split" is involved. In other words, if the dedicated professionals cannot achieve consensus on what Cartesian dualism means, there is far less of a chance that the much looser and more dramatic version has any single coherent meaning. And yet the phrase is almost always presented with this apparent assumption, without any accompanying explication. It seems to be just-so, and yet, on closer inspection, it seems to disappear, like a tantalizing mirage. This is what I mean by the Cartesian Split being nowhere.

As such, I believe it to be best to start with an empty mind. Perhaps we may learn anew, from this survey, what this phrase actually signifies, in its current use. Extending the therapeutic analogy, what I am attempting here is a kind of word association test, performed on our subject Ash. By starting with a survey of abstracts and titles in this way, I am essentially opening the session by asking: "What is the first thing you think of when I say 'Cartesian Split?'" At this point, the task of therapist is to document Ash's story fully, without stopping to question for veracity.

Although the final result of this survey reflects a very wide range of material, there are a few generic and repeated themes, which can be used to organize the results. These categories are certainly not rigid; there is a significant amount of overlap between them, but they are still a useful starting point. For each of these categories or themes, I will generally start with the material from the word association test, that is, the survey of abstracts and title only. I will then, as therapist, ask for more detail. To do this, I will draw in material from other sources, to further illustrate and amplify the themes found by this initial word association.

For all sources, I will often be explicit, citing as much original text as needed. This is not to save me the effort of writing, rather, it is important to capture the essence of the material. In general, I focus on commentary with unusually strong and dramatic language, which is a good indicator of a psychological complex at work. Often, it is the precise choice of words that can reveal the deeper meaning, which would be lost if I were to paraphrase the source.

Although the goal of the chapter is to document the voice of the complex fully, without unnecessary critique or judgment, I will conclude each section with some brief commentary and evaluation, to highlight certain problems, such as inconsistencies and ironies. This is such that the complex can become more aware of itself as a complex, and less of a rote analysis of the history of ideas. This complex is a product of the imagination, and I mean this in a positive way. The imagination should be recognized and valued for what it uniquely offers, and from this, we may be able to imagine a solution.

Body as machine

One of the more prevalent themes is what may be termed the "body-as-machine" metaphor. This would be the view that, under the influence of the Cartesian Split, personal identity is divided into a living mind and a mechanical body. However, the emphasis is more on the development of the latter conception as a dominant worldview and the limitations that this presents.

In the survey of abstracts, I found many of these references come from academic areas related to the health professions. Several argue that this metaphor has led to various unfortunate practices in Western medicine. This includes the misuse of psychotropic medicine (Kellogg, 2013), the improper diagnosis of "brain-dead" (Lock, 2002), inadequate ways of talking about pain (Bendelow, 2006) and risk (Kavanagh & Broom, 1998). Others have discussed ways in which the body-as-machine metaphor has limited Western medicine in general (Brencick, 1997; Thayer, 2009).

Again, in these abstracts, the exact meaning of these invocations is not entirely clear. Fortunately, I believe the overall sentiment is well reflected in cell biologist Bruce Lipton's (2008) bestseller, *The Biology of Belief*. In this work, Descartes is shown to be foundational to the development of a mechanistic view in biomedicine, in which the mind has no influence (pp. 94–95). As the patient-body is seen only as a machine, critical opportunities are missed or neglected. By focusing on the healing power of the mind, Lipton hopes to enhance medicine, by re-uniting "Science and Spirit." "These realms were split apart in the days of Descartes centuries ago" (p. 155). It is interesting to note here Lipton's attitude when compared to the neuroscientist Damasio. Both are scientists who resent Descartes' residual influence but argue against it in two very divergent directions. Lipton challenges it in order to rediscover the mind, over and above the machine body. But for Damasio, it is to marginalize the rational mind and to focus more on the importance of the bodily emotions.

In another work, the body-as-machine metaphor is construed in a rather dark light, bordering on existential dread. For Lloyd (2011), "the Cartesian body" simply goes about its motions in a cold, dull and lifeless manner. It has "lost its foundational connection to the vital breath as well as the animate world" (p. 76). In this account, there is a clear call to see the body as more than just a lifeless machine, to see human beings as more than just a lump of meat.

These modern accounts have a surprising analogue to a common folk-tale about Descartes, told in the 18th through 20th centuries. In these stories, according to Gaukroger (1998), Descartes was rumored to always be accompanied with a mechanical replica of his illegitimate daughter, Francine. He was even rumored to have slept with it by his side. Those who saw the doll were horrified by such a "mechanical monstrosity," and were compelled to get rid of it (p. 1).

Of course, according to Gaukroger (1998), "there is no evidence that any version of the story is true." Instead, it appears to be a subsequently developed propaganda piece, developed not so much against Descartes, but against La Mettrie's 18th-century treatise *L'Homme Machine* (p. 1). La Mettrie's account, for those who are not familiar, is actually much closer to the materialism currently in our health sciences. And so, evidently, the propaganda has survived for centuries, all the while retaining a curious mismatch between names and theories. In any case, it is firmly believed today that "Cartesian" is equated with a kind of soulless materialism.

It is true that Descartes explicitly compared animals to machines, often regarded as the "infamous" *Bête-machine* doctrine, although it has been significantly misinterpreted and misunderstood. This will be explored more in the subsequent chapters. Regardless, this doctrine has its own share of exaggerated tales, and many of these are in academic works, even recent ones. According to Forsman (2015), in one account, Descartes is said to have kicked a pregnant dog and explained its whimpers as nothing more than mere automatic expressions of a machine. In another legend, he "nailed his wife's dog to a board plank for vivisection" in order to prove to her it was a machine. Again, none of these tales have any direct evidence of historical truth. In some cases, the details are in direct conflict to the known facts of the historical Descartes (para. 1–3).

This has, of course, not stopped the vitality of the legend. According to Rupert Sheldrake (2012), Descartes had a test for would-be followers, being required to kick their own dogs, in order to prove their acceptance of his machine model (pp. 32–33). What is curious about this instance is that Sheldrake provides a direct reference to Descartes' writings, giving it the appearance of authenticity. Upon inspection, however, the source text has no details of this kind. Evidently, the legend just *feels* so true that the tale jumps off of an otherwise routine page during research, and into the author's imagination, as a self-evident interpretation. Perhaps it is not enough to say that Descartes' reputation precedes him. The reputation precedes him by such a large degree that it has become its own reality, perhaps "hyperreal," as Baudrillard might say.

Ecological crisis

Scholars focusing on environmental studies see the Cartesian Split as more far-ranging, and particularly destructive, in large-scale ecological systems. In the abstracts, Storm (2015) implicates the Cartesian split in both environmental destruction and our ability to even properly describe it. Mortimore (2013) sees the split as that which forcefully maintains a lifestyle that prevents traditional ecological living, leading to global ecological ruin. Similarly, Fenwick (1998) suggests the Cartesian split has restricted theoretical models in ecopsychology from addressing important environmental issues.

The sentiment is certainly echoed in other, dedicated works in ecopsychology. Gary Snyder (2001), a widely recognized leader in the field, states that the work of Descartes, along with Newton and Hobbes, amounted to a "profound rejection of the organic world." As a result, the "occidental scientist-engineer-ruler puts the whole planet on the brink of degradation" (pp. 18–19). David Abram (2002), writing in the foreword of Andy Fisher's *Radical Ecopsychology*, starts immediately, in the first two paragraphs, in familiar Cartesian terrain. "Ever since the Enlightenment, technological civilization has assumed a clear divide" between two worlds. It is an "age-old divide between mind and matter, between the psyche 'in here' and nature 'out there.'" This split has taken "a tremendous toll. . . on the animate earth around us" (p. ix).

In Abram's (1997) own book, *The Spell of the Sensuous*, he takes up the topic again, this time explicitly tying it to Descartes. Conveniently, he also brings in the machine metaphor, which has its source in "Descartes's well-known separation" of mind and matter (pp. 31–32). The separation, it must be emphasized was deeply tragic to the earlier, more inclusive worldview. "In Descartes's hands. . . this hierarchical continuum of living forms, commonly called 'the Great Chain of Being,' was polarized into a thorough dichotomy between mechanical, unthinking matter" and mind (p. 48). What followed from this was a justification to exploit nature for our own use. It was a "splendid rationalization for the vivisection experiments that soon began to proliferate, as well as for the steady plundering and despoilment of nonhuman nature" (pp. 77–78).

Another example is from Kureethadam's (2017) *The Philosophical Roots of the Ecological Crisis*, which is subtitled: *Descartes and the Modern Worldview*. The reason for this subtitle is that all previous attempts to trace these roots are found wanting, neglecting the single, especially pernicious root that is Descartes (p. 4). Notably, the stakes of the crisis are high. It is "not just the survival of many forms of life but the very future of human civilization" (p. 1). Facing the crisis requires an in-depth challenging of the modern worldview, which has three components: An exaggerated anthropocentrism, the machine model, and metaphysical dualism. These three prongs "can all be largely traced back to the Cartesian thought with direct ecological consequences" (p. 5).

In a recent online article, Taylor Steelman (2018) considers the "Cartesian self" to be directly opposed to ecological living. Worse, according to another author, Daniel Quinn, it is "the most dangerous thing in existence—more dangerous than our all nuclear armaments, more dangerous than biological warfare, more dangerous than all the pollutants we pump into the air, the water, and the land" (para. 1). Further, "colonialism, slavery, and capitalism — these are all legacies of the Cartesian self" (para. 7). But ecology, given the high stakes, is the ultimate concern. "Western civilization, under command of the Cartesian self, is the meteor causing the Sixth Mass Extinction on planet Earth" (para. 11).

All of the preceding claims are certainly concerning, given the potential implications. By referring to such claims as evidence of a complex, as products of the imagination, I do not intend to belittle or falsify those concerns. Personally, I do accept that there is an ecological crisis, and I also fully support the need to study it in the context of the history of ideas. But for this to happen, we need to be very precise with our understanding of the ideas themselves. The history of ideas is enormously complex, with very large challenges, such as minding interpretation, translations, and context. This is a task normally reserved for dedicated scholars of philosophy. By contrast, these sources are from outside this field, and these challenges are usually not confronted. Rather, they are replaced with an unusual amount of confidence and accompanied by rather strong language. This is one reason to consider such commentary as part of a complex. In summation, there may indeed be an ecological crisis, but the language used to describe it suggests there is yet another meaning to it.

Feminist challenge

Although critiques are found across a wide range of disciplines, the ones from a feminist background deserve special mention. This particular angle was a salient feature in at least three places in the initial survey. In Vertinsky's (2001) paper, which features feminism in the title, it is suggested that a certain feminist theorist's career trajectory is best encapsulated by her challenges to the Cartesian split, which is partly to blame for harmful gender roles. Orning (2012) notes a similar relationship. Beginning with the goal of a "non-Cartesian subject," she emphasizes two contemporary works of fiction, featuring "female, literary freaks," that exemplify this goal. Similarly, Mortimore brings a "feminist, arts-informed inquiry" to the global industrial crisis, which is notably maintained by the Cartesian split. Similar sentiments are found in Kavanagh and Broom (1998) and Fisanick (2003).

From a wider review of material, it is clear that feminist studies take an unusually strong interest in the legacy of Descartes. In some cases, such a legacy is not only suggested to impede the goals of feminism, but is believed to be harmful, or actively misogynistic, even in our own times. For example, Cortesi (2013) finds Cartesian dualism to be an active presence in romance novels, in spite of its having been discredited in academia. Under its influence, the heroines' minds, because they are separate, are unable to stop their bodies from submitting to sexual violence. In other words, their minds say no, but it does not matter, because their bodies say yes. For Orr (2007), a similar feeling is found in a different context. After some surgeries in Western medicine, she writes that "my body had been well and truly partitioned by the medical profession and its Cartesian language" (p. 103). In both cases, it is striking to see a ghost of a philosophical legacy inhabiting women's bodies against their will.

There are many other related examples scattered across modern academic feminism. It is enough to have prompted Sorell (2005) to dedicate an entire section of his book on Descartes on it, subtitled "Cartesian Misogyny?" (pp. 141–148). Further, Bordo (1999) edited and wrote the introduction for an anthology titled *Feminist Interpretations of René Descartes*, which includes many sentiments echoing this theme. It is possible that most of these works stem from the seminal work by Genevieve Lloyd (1993), originally published in 1984, titled "The Man of Reason." In this book, it is argued that Descartes effectively ushered in a certain masculinization of thought, or as Lloyd calls a "sexual division of mental labour." In short, women are relegated to the realm of the irrational body, from which the "Cartesian Man of Reason must transcend" (pp. 50–51). It is clear from this that some of feminism's favorite topics, such as phallocentric thinking, the hegemony of reason, and the marginalization of the body and other forms of non-rationality, are all closely aligned with Lloyd's critique.

However, like all good complex material, things are more complex the further you investigate. Even in Lloyd's own work, she is somewhat ambivalent if the blame can be placed so neatly in one source. She recognizes that the separation of mind from body can, in principle, lead to a non-gendered way of thinking. Also, the lack of gender in some of Descartes' writings invites women to participate in the philosophical discussion. Given this understanding, Lloyd suggests that his writings may have had the unfortunate and opposite effect of his own intentions. Bordo (1999), in her introduction to the anthology noted above, also takes care to note the subtlety and seeming contradiction in these arguments. However, it seems that most feminist critiques have lost this subtlety, and maintain the Cartesian dualism is inherently and wholly anti-feminist.

Subjective difficulties

Two works in this initial survey seem to suggest that the Cartesian split is more problematic at the subjective level, rather than with anything specifically regarding the body or the environment. Hollomon (2000), writing in the field of psychotherapy, states that the split has rendered the self unable to relate to "Truth." It is only through challenging and transcending the split that "enlightened subjective self-awareness" is made possible. In legal scholarship, Pether (1999) argues that prominent theory in the field is flawed on account of poor self-awareness, complicated by the "Cartesian split subject."

It may not be clear what these authors are intending exactly, but in other works, there are some direct associations to some kind of subject-level psychopathology, and this is essentially how I am attempting to capture this theme. For example, for Fisher (2002), Cartesian dualism is not so much about two different substances, but rather, it "describes only self-estranged, disembodied, narcissistic experience" (p. 56). Or, the Cartesian search for foundations is symptomatic of an unhealthy and unnatural anxiety (p. 121). Berman (1981) compares Descartes' mechanical model of the body to schizophrenia. "This schizoid duality lies at the heart of the Cartesian paradigm" (p. 35). For Bray and Colebrook (1998), "the Cartesian cogito is paranoid and narcissistic" (p. 40). For Bateson (2000), Cartesian dualism is to blame for an alcoholic's inability to admit their own addiction (p. 313). Potter (2011), through the work of Laing, looks at the "Cartesian shadow as returning symptomatically as cultural psychosis and individual afflictions of normal alienation and schizophrenic alienation" (p. 11). For Atwood, Stolorow and Orange (2011), Cartesianism represents a pathological view of the mind as being self-existing and autonomous, and this is a "form of madness—a Cartesian madness—that splits asunder the unbroken, organic unity of life and thought" (p. 265).

Finally, Charles Pope (2011) describes a "Cartesian Anxiety," in which the mind suffers in isolation, disconnected from the body and all of reality. This mind suffers from anxiety because it tries to rely on itself for an absolute foundation of truth, but tragically, cannot. It also leads to an imbalance, "between certainty and doubt, faith and reason, body and mind" (para. 2). Curiously, the first two of these pairs of opposites are within the mind, while the third features mind as only one side.

All of the above examples are rather unusual ways of understanding Cartesian philosophy. After all, "I think, therefore I am" is perhaps the most well-known and famous statement of subjective self-awareness, a clarion call for clear-headed rationalism. It is, in fact, the very definition of rationalism, in the philosophical tradition, that the mind can retreat into itself and find within it everything it needs to find truth. Perhaps this move is somewhat incomplete or problematic in context, but its essential meaning is that the subjective thinking process itself is working properly. And so, it is indeed odd to now see this basic meaning of the most famous line from such a famous philosopher completely inverted.

Over-rationality

In the abstracts, two works present a related theme, in that they focus on the problem of the mind being split off from a larger, fuller experience, although still internally healthy. In other words, the mind creates problems by doing too much of what it does well. The mind also takes on more of the meaning of an intellectual, rational mind, rather than thinking in general. In anthropology, Goodrich (2004) states that the split invalidly privileges rationality, and thereby "disqualifies spatial knowledge," or that which is related to the body. This situation is "fundamentally alienating." In a journal on public administration, Isaacs (2001) states that the "instrumental rationality" of the Cartesian split has historically frustrated effective works. Through the practice of dialogue, which is outside of the control of the intellect, "unrealized levels of coordination and insight" may yet be realized.

The same sentiment is found in other works. For Wilde (2013), "Cartesian thinking" is a dangerous artifact of the mathematical, industrial age. If left alone, it can lure us into a state of "an existential human sense of lack, a grasping mode," which prevents "a sense of completeness and peace" (p. 29). Balzac (2008) sees the various "Cartesian Splits" whenever an intellectually gifted child gets frustrated from not being able to apply their intelligence to athletics. For Pope John Paul II, writing with Messori (1994), Descartes is the central figure in the rationalism of the Enlightenment, but this is seen as an overwhelmingly negative development. This is because the final result of rationalism is an excessive scientific secularism, with God being "expelled from the world," being only an "unverifiable hypothesis" (p. 53).

All of these works are essentially recapitulating Damasio's argument. That is, Descartes's error was not so much concerning mind itself, rather only in privileging the rational, intellectual mind, over and above the body. As a neuroscientist, Damasio surely appreciates rationality, and further, his tools of investigation could not have even existed without the infamous machine model in medicine. But what is most interesting about this overall sentiment is the breadth of its scope. A neuroscientist and the Pope may not have much in common, but at least they can agree on one thing, that Descartes' rationality distances us from what matters the most. For one, it is the body, for the other, God.

Limitations in expression

In the initial survey, I found several works in fields inclined toward the humanities, in which it is seen that the Cartesian split has frustrated our ability to effectively write and express ourselves. For Washburn (2012), it is has led to trends in academic writing which is "devoid of pathos and lacking true ethos." In this work, which is titled "Healing the Cartesian Split," the author also endorses Damasio as at least a partial solution. For Mkhatshwa (2010), the split has dislocated authorial intention, which may lead to problems with interpretation and transparency. For Smith (2015), the split is the basis for the "dominant perceptive regimen" which is preventing "radical new types of spatial construction." For Orning (2012), the historical split is evaluated in the arts, and this legacy is proclaimed to have led to invalid and unhealthy standards of what is normal for the human body. Metzger (1987), writing on missionary work, sees narration as an effective solution to the various problems raised by the split. In education, it is suggested that teachers are limited because the Cartesian split "demands" that they ignore their bodies (Fisanick, 2003). In the field of science, technology, and human values, the split has limited the effectiveness of artistic representation (Hoeppe, 2015).

In other works, Potter (2011) opens up a study on the sublime with a rather stark vision. The "Cartesian linear perspective" is ultimately self-destructive and renders it nearly impossible to retain the aesthetics of the humanities. "Aesthetic elements of the sublime have been eclipsed under the sway of a particularly Cartesian stance pressing the isolated ego against the cold, dead world of matter" (p. 1). Similarly, for Temple-Hoon (2012), James Hillman's aesthetic approach "reinvigorates the relationship between the soul and its images by waking imagination from its Cartesian slumber" (p. 11). It has also hindered the ability of black Christians to fully express bodily sensuality in worship, because they remain caught in the "Cartesian captivity" of the split (Dyson, 2001, p. 317). But it is not just the humanities that are being held back. According to Newell, as cited in Güzeldere and Franchi (1995), the Cartesian split is responsible for the disbelief in the future success of Artificial Intelligence (para. 4).

Again, anti-Cartesianism is a wide net, welcoming in champions of both the arts and technology. And so, it is fitting to find another critique from a study of Japanese anime, which often blends those ideals together, particularly with its frequent portrayals of cyborgs. For Tomos (2013), Hollywood is dominated and restricted by its "Cartesian duality," but anime successfully breaks from this limitation (p. 314). Also, a leading figure in the field, Oshii, "challenged the Cartesian perspective of the division of body and soul," and by this, a humanistic portrayal of cyborgs is made possible (p. 282).

If it were true that the Cartesian Split is responsible for holding back artistic expression, it would be ironic to note instances in which the Split itself is featured in works of art. I have found two such instances. According to an online description of a 1993 art exhibit, artists Conway and Pratt (2019) have created a multimedia exhibit titled "The Elevated Examination of the Cartesian Split." As best as I can tell, the piece featured audio of a disembodied voice, a man coldly describing his surroundings in a "hapless" elevator ride. Also, I found an audio recording, titled "Cartesian Split," credited to Koopman (2019), which starts off with highly dramatic notes, not unlike something found in a scene from a horror movie. Interestingly, the piece ends with some rather calm, melodic progressions. Perhaps this is an artistic attempt at a resolution to a now well-known philosophical tragedy. In any case, from a broad view, it appears that Cartesian Split both hinders art and inspires it at the same time. Such a bipolar evaluation of a single subject is another distinguishing feature of a complex.

Reduction and isolation

One prevalent conception is that the Cartesian split harms us by imposing a restrictive, reductive worldview of isolated parts, rather than of synergistic wholes. This is related to the body-as-machine metaphor but has more to do with mechanistic reductionism in general.

In the survey of abstracts, various other conceptions of relationship or holism are offered as a needed alternative, such as our "intrinsic interconnection" (Bright, 2015), relational systems models in developmental psychology, pointing the way to a "post-Cartesian" era (Overton, 2013), and activities "reuniting the Cartesian split" to bring back a "sense of wholeness" (Maddock & Humphries, 2010). Rosado (2008) sees the breakdown into parts as extending across virtually every field of human culture. "We live in a divided world dominated by a fragmentary worldview," which has been "fuelled" by the Cartesian Split.

In other works, Brady (1977) defines Cartesianism as "the felt alienation of mind from extended bodies," featured in the detached, objective scientific observer. By removing the observer from the observation, reality becomes a dead machine, mindlessly executing the laws of nature. The result is that the "universe is devoid of consciousness, empty of mind" (pp. 2–3). By contrast, holistic thinking challenges the "mechanistic discreteness that structures the Cartesian view" (p. 14). For Ponte and Schäfer (2013), Descartes' declarations, along with Newton and Darwin, directly led to a "totalitarian materialistic environment," where "anything that wasn't matter didn't matter." In this deterministic environment, there are only individual particles competing for dominance, with no sense of mutual interconnection (p. 602).

Perhaps Whitehead's (1938) *Modes of Thought* was the first to take up this anti-positivistic stance, and quite poignantly. "The scientific world is suffering from a bad attack of muddle-headed positivism" in which nature is nothing but chemical processes. Also, "the whole doctrine of life in nature has suffered from this positivist taint," and this developed directly from Cartesian dualism. "The effect of this sharp division between nature and life has poisoned all subsequent philosophy" (p. 204). Further, "Science can find no individual enjoyment in nature: Science can find no aim in nature: Science can find no creativity in nature; it finds mere rules of succession" (p. 211).

This sentiment is likely behind the prevalent misunderstanding of Descartes' conception of God. It is common to assume that since the Cartesian universe is nothing but clockwork, then the Cartesian God is nothing but a clockmaker, who, after the initial winding up the clock, is no longer necessary. In short, God is "expendable" (Stern, 1999, p. 45), merely an observer, limited to watching the playing out of these rules of succession. This portrayal is far from accurate, as Descartes' God is continuously creating and sustaining the universe.

Overall, however, I can sympathize with many of these positions, having in my own personal life a period of profound dissatisfaction with excessive scientism, and I also attributed this to Descartes. But I also realized in my reflections, that I was once entranced and enthralled with these "mere rules" of natural science. Such a re-evaluation can also be found in an empathetic reading of the history of science. In the 17th and 18th centuries, scientific luminaries were excited and enthusiastic about the new mechanical philosophy sweeping across Europe, because they enabled so many new discoveries and technologies. The notion of *reducing* phenomena to something more dull and banal would have been unthinkable to them. Perhaps, then, this overall shift in attitude could be understood as simply the lifecycle of a paradigm. However, this could be applied to any paradigm, not just classical mechanics. To my knowledge, we do not levy so much harsh blame on every outdated founder of every paradigm. Descartes get disproportional blame in this regard, and this is what matters for this study.

Pairs of opposites

As stated, one peculiar characteristic of the Cartesian Split is its unusually wide scope. In the following summary of references from the field of abstracts, this is demonstrated in wide variety of different pairs of opposites. Of course, all of them problematic or invalid, and must be rejected.

The Cartesian split is either between the observer and the "other" (Lapointe, 1976), mind versus body, nature versus nurture, psychological versus social (Cushman, 2011), soma versus psyche (Bankart, 2006), or material versus mental (Shapiro, 2015). In the previously mentioned works, the split also occurs in mind versus world (Fenwick, 1998), body versus self (Kavanagh & Broom, 1998), spatial knowledge versus practical consciousness (Goodrich, 2004), pathos versus academic writing (Washburn, 2012), consciousness versus being (Mkhatshwa, 2010), normal versus abnormal (Orning, 2012), inner versus outer (Bright, 2015), bodies versus teaching (Fisanick, 2003), experience of aging versus conceptions of aging (Goebel, 2014), experience versus physical reality (Brencick, 1997), knower versus known (Hollomon, 2000), and finally, heaven versus Earth, and nature versus culture (Mortimore, 2013). Fittingly, Rosado (2008) characterizes the Cartesian split as an "either/or understanding of reality."

From other sources, a particularly strong exhibit of this comes from a book review by Lerner (1999), another work titled "Healing the Cartesian Split." In this work, there is an impressive display of long lists of paired opposites, which might be seen as a Cartesian Split "run." In the opening paragraph alone, the Cartesian Split is framed as between continuity versus discontinuity, stability versus instability, constancy versus change, nature versus nurture. Further, the latter by itself manifests in many other forms, namely "maturation-experience; inborn-learned; heredity-environment; innate-acquired; organism-environment; person-context; gene-environment; and organicism-mechanism." Naturally, it is then suspected that the entire enterprise is flawed on account of an illegitimate "either/or" way of thinking (para. 1–2), which of course is shared by Rosado. These latter two perspectives nicely summarize this entire survey of pairs of opposites. In other words, anything that can be conceived in the frame of a logical opposition is automatically suspect, due to the presupposed Cartesian split underlying and infecting them all.

More splits of different kinds, and more patterns of splits, may be found in other works as well. In one example, the Cartesian Split is between man and woman, and even between black and white (Reid-Pharr, 1999, p. 45). Maguire (1997) sees "the Cartesian revolution" as causing "the rupture between science and wisdom" (p. 69). Skrbina (2007) is not content with defining Cartesian dualism in only one pair. Descartes is in fact was a "double-dualist," the first dualism being ontological, between mind and matter, and the second categorical, between mindful humans versus a mindless universe (p. 387). Smith (1985), in a review of Bernstein, follows Rosado in the more generic form of a Cartesian "either/or," but it becomes more dramatic. "Cartesian Anxiety" is defined by the "grand Either/Or," which is explained as an "unbearable tension between *either* finding support for truth, *or* succumbing to madness and chaos" (p. 61). For Lovejoy (1955), the split, which has for most of history been "unchallengeable," is between the knower and the known, experience and nature, and mental from the physical (p. 3), and is also the "bifurcation of nature" into subjective and objective (p. 4). For Temple-Hoon (2012), split is between "subject and the object, the mind and the body, and immanence and transcendence" (p. 7), and as another "either/or" (p. 11). For Bateson (2000), if we continue with Cartesian dualism, we will eventually see the world in terms of "God versus man; elite versus people; chosen race versus others; nation versus nation; and man versus environment" (p. 337). Kelso (2015) defines the Cartesian Split as "that fateful division that now dominates all branches of knowledge," manifesting as a split between "head/heart, conscious/unconscious, within/without, here/there, this/that, and body/mind" (para. 2). For Seidl (2013), the split is "the division between mind and body, reason and intuition" (para 3), and may also be associated with the two hemispheres of the brain. But biology is not necessarily a hindrance, as the work can be done with good philosophy: "Let's heal this split, I say, be it between the hemispheres or between reason/analysis and body/intuition" (para 4).

In one curious example, I found an article for an architecture journal, titled "The Cartesian Split," attributed to Spuybroek (1999). I was not able to read the entire article, so I could not get the proper context, but on the page viewable to me, there was a hand-drawn schematic that featured a wide array of opposites, with "The Cartesian Split" prominently in the middle. These pairs were Europe-America, Floor-Wall, Program-Form, Action-Perception, Plan-Elevation, and Feet-Eyes (p. 13).

Avens (1988) follows Lerner with three different runs, all on one page, or a run of runs. Cartesian influence is first established as the "double curse" of the West, and this manifests as a split between "the unlimited and the limited, the eternal and the temporal, spirit and matter." Then, new ideas are needed in order to reunite "the spiritual and the physical, the divine and the human, the universal and the concrete." Finally, with the right perspective, "the question of 'inner' and 'outer,' subjective and objective, spirit and matter, simply does not arise" (p. 382).

The dominant paradigm

In the collection of abstracts, several works strike a somewhat epochal tone in the framing of the Cartesian Split. The sense is that the Split is so dominant and so widespread that you have to take a long, historical view, in order to solve the real problem. It is also necessarily assumed the Split is part of a dominant worldview that is highly resistant to challenge. For Lerner (1999), the various splits in developmental psychology have resulted in "literally hundreds of empirical investigations" that have not made any progress toward their goals. For Maddock and Humphries (2010), the western worldview, now being challenged, dominates us "with an intense and far-reaching grip." For Marshall (2015), the "Cartesian-Split-Mechanistic approach" has been "historically imposed" on us, limiting future progress. Silverstein (2003) writes a historical study and notes "the Cartesian Split, the prevailing paradigm," which may be preventing nursing from entering the 21st century.

It is not altogether surprising to find such examples, as Descartes is widely known as the "father of modern philosophy." But in other examples, what stands out is the degree of this particular father's influence, and how truly strong and pervasive it is. For Barron (2015), "echoes of Descartes's dualism" can be found in not just prominent modern philosophers, but can "be discerned, as well, in the speech and attitudes of millions of ordinary people today" (para 3). For Brady (1981), shortly after Aquinas, "the rise of nominalism would lay the groundwork of the Cartesian split, and the premise of the separation of mind and object would hypnotize Western thought for several hundred years" (p. 5). For Graffman (2017) "most of our everyday thinking and 'science' still contends with the physicalist strictures laid down by Descartes," and we are "plagued by it daily" (p. 147). Finally, Whitehead (1938) continues his lament against scientism by invoking its notorious founder. "The disastrous separation of body and mind which has been fixed on European thought by Descartes is responsible for this blindness of Science" (p. 211).

Descartes is also a is a favorite figure to mark as a pivotal point in history, a certain founding father of the modern age. This extends into specific fields as well, including psychology. Makari (2009) begins his history of psychoanalysis with Descartes (p. 9), and Jung follows suit, with his history of psychology in general (Hannah, 1976, p. 217). Overall, he represents a convenient and comforting way to divide history into stages, and for this reason, it is common to portray him as a sort of revolutionary, radical figure (Baker & Morris, 2002, p. 3). Unfortunately, as these authors and others have demonstrated, this turns out to be a vast oversimplification. Descartes' actual writings indicate he was actually quite traditional and conservative in many respects (Ariew, 1992).

In many other examples, the same sentiment appears, but now with Descartes in concert with other historical figures. Lipton (2008), who is particularly fond of blaming Descartes, also takes the time to implicate Copernicus and Darwin in the tragic "Spirit/Science split" (p. 157). For Abram (1997), Copernicus, Galileo, Kepler also get the blame for "a profound schism. . . between our intellectual convictions and the most basic conviction of our senses." But fittingly, after this he seems compelled to mention Descartes in a parenthetical (pp. 42–43). For de Quincey (2008), it was not until Whitehead that we had a way out of the "Cartesian-Kantian impasse" (p. 2). For Lovejoy (1955), it is the "the Age of the Great Revolt against Dualism," but this "uprising" is against both Galileo and Descartes, who together have "bound the minds of reflective men, and especially men of science, ever since" (p. 1). For Capra (1983), the names Descartes and Newton are used almost interchangeably, but when one is needed as a target, it is almost always the "Cartesian world view" (pp. 15–16). For these and many others, Descartes is both *the* father, and at the same time, just one of many fathers.

In spite of this, for most others, Descartes singularly retains the title of the "father" of modern philosophy, and we also have the common presupposition that modern consciousness today is thoroughly "Cartesian." However, dedicated Cartesian scholars are quick to note that this is a problematic understanding. Historically, Descartes' work did find a few early adherents but was also met with fierce rejection and criticism from authorities, including church, state, and universities. In 1663, his works were even placed on the *List of Prohibited Books* (Jolley, 1992, p. 398). The few who did appreciate some of the core ideas, such as Spinoza and Leibniz, generally developed them in very different directions (p. 412), and to such an extent that it is debatable if even they can be called Cartesian. By the time Cartesian influence gained any kind of a foothold, it was quickly superseded by Newton's in physics, and by Locke's in philosophy (p. 419). A complementary history is documented by Carolyn Merchant (as Iltis, 1973). For these reasons, many philosophers note the irony of this overall claim by putting "father" in quotes.

For some, Cartesianism is strangely both pervasive and absent at the same time. Koestler (1964) states that the Cartesian spirit mostly died out on the continent, but survived the longest in France, until the second half of the 19th century, until Charcot (p. 152). But just two pages later, he argues that the Cartesian tradition is alive and well, "deeply engrained in our thinking habits" (p. 154). Similarly, Whitehead (1979) states that "we no more retain the physics of the seventeenth century than we do the Cartesian philosophy of that century" (p. 14), in spite of also emphatically blaming the current "blindness of science" on Descartes, as cited earlier. Whitehead is similarly conflicted on the value of the ideas themselves. On one hand, we owe to Descartes a "disastrous separation of body and mind." On the other, "Descartes undoubtedly made the greatest philosophical discovery since the age of Plato and Aristotle" (p. 159).

Old versus new

Still, for most, the Cartesian paradigm is believed to be dominant and has been so for centuries. In spite of this daunting historical backdrop, many of the abstracts feature a hopeful tone, concerning some new development, which offers a potential solution to the age-old crisis. For this, new ideas are sought for in some perhaps unlikely places. Some of the more noteworthy fields, mined for such inspiration, include shamanism (Thayer, 2009), Buddhism (Bankart, 2006), systems theory (Shapiro, 2015), and quantum physics (Maddock & Humphries, 2010). Of course, the first two are not new, but perhaps new to the average Western reader, and this is what seems to count. It is not really necessary to provide any more details to this theme, as it is naturally implied by all sources mentioned thus far. To dedicate such effort toward rejecting the old Cartesian worldview is to necessarily assume something novel to replace it, if only the author's own writing.

There is also a certain socialization move implied by these claims. Lee (2013) describes a certain "Cartesian complex," which is the fear that an academic might be described by another as being Cartesian (pp. 85–86). The dividing line is always clear. To be new and exciting, you have to be able to demonstrate your emancipation from the old Cartesian ways.

What is most interesting about this particular move is that, every time it is invoked, "Cartesian" must be framed as a singular thing, an old thing, and this is starkly opposed to something radically new. In other words, *either* you are mired in the old Cartesian ways, *or* you are with the new and the sophisticated. But we have also learned that anything framed as an either/or proposition *is itself Cartesian*. The Cartesian Split is truly everywhere, and now it is fractal and scale-free. From this way of thinking, it can never be overcome.

Heroic transcenders

Frequently, in the context of presenting a new idea to challenge the split, a particular theorist or other noteworthy figure is presented as an especially heroic figure. The story of this hero usually requires the theme of the Dominant Paradigm. In other words, it is a better story if everyone else is stuck in the thrall of the Cartesian Split, except for the one lone heroic figure who has managed to challenge it.

This theme appeared prominently in the survey of abstracts. For Vertinsky (2001), this figure is Charlotte Gilman, who is celebrated for her "breakaway from the accepted medical paradigm based on the Cartesian split," and for her offering of a "radically new mind/body concept." For Marshall (2015) a similar figure is found in Sporn, whose work on embodiment offers a way out of the dead ends "imposed" by the split. For Brencick (1997), the hero is herself. She writes, "I overcome the Cartesian split," by demonstrating that the body-as-machine view is impossible. For Bright (2015), if we follow Jung's lead, "outdated dualistic thinking. . . can be demolished." For Fenwick, the "split between mind and world" calls for a new paradigm in our "whole way of thinking," and this may be found in the work of Mindell. Goebel (2014) celebrates Amery, who "bridges the abyss," and is led to a "convincing rethinking of the Cartesian split." For LaPointe (1976), Merleau-Ponty's views oppose the split, which is found in Sartre. For Orning (2012), writers Dunn and Carter are noted because "they refuse the Cartesian split," that which has been in place since the 17th century.

The theme appears in many other sources as well. In fact, upon collecting so many exhibits, I was struck at how many times the Cartesian Split has already been solved. There should, in fact, be no reason for me to write this book, because for some, the error was corrected as soon as it was released on an unsuspecting world. For example, Voltaire (1901), writing in the 18th century, chastises Descartes' description of the soul as being distinct from the body. In response, he celebrates Locke, the "one truly wise man" who has finally corrected this error and "given us its real history," showing to man "the anatomy of his own soul" (pp. 35–36). In more recent commentary, a contemporary to Locke is also celebrated. For Thayer (1919), Spinoza, in his final days, intends to correct Descartes' conceptions before he dies. His goal in this is nothing less than the reunification of God and extension (p. 97). Perhaps at about the same time, Swedenborg was coming along, a rare talent indeed. He shared with the mystics a "dual vision," a master of the two worlds, and this gave him the "difficult and unpopular task of resuscitating the soul as the third realm between matter and spirit" (Avens, 1988, p. 382).

The following century also had its fair share of heroic transcenders. Hume, following Locke, finally "completes the breakdown of Cartesian metaphysics," but even goes further, by "destroy[ing] the ground for the Cartesian explanation of a mind to its own ideas" (Watson, 1998, p. 130). And yet, it was left to Kant to provide a "thoroughgoing critique of Descartes' subjectivism, and destroys the Cartesian barrier" (Schwyzer, 1997).

In the early 19th century, the battle was being joined on another front, by various luminaries in science. For according to Capra (1983), it was Faraday and Maxwell as the "first to go beyond" classical mechanics (p. 70), which for Capra, is virtually synonymous with Cartesianism. There was also the fatal blow dealt by Darwin's theory of evolution, which "forced scientists to abandon the Cartesian conception" of mechanism (p. 72). Finally, Stumpf praises Helmholtz for his singular efforts to "bridge the gulf between Physiology and Psychology—a bridge across which thousands of other men now constantly come and go" (as cited by Makari, 2009, p. 68).

Many other heroes are found in the late 19th century. William James's radical empiricism did not just "attack" Hegelian absolute idealism, but also "broke sharply" with dualism as well. In order "to transcend this Cartesian dualism," he now proposed pure experience as the fundamental reality (Smith, 2015). Meanwhile, back on the continent, Husserl was becoming frustrated by the mathematizing influence of Galileo and Descartes, which forced him to "inaugurate" the field of phenomenology, in order to rescue and preserve the world of immediate experience (Abram, 1997, p. 35). And yet, strangely enough, Husserl had heroic company with two famous British mathematicians. For Lovejoy (1955) it was Whitehead who has done more than anyone else to reject dualism, the "bifurcation of nature," in Whitehead's owns terms. Thus, Whitehead brings forth a new philosophy, one "radically different," and becomes "one of the major prophets" of the new school of objective realism (pp. 193–194). But Whitehead had help from a close associate, for it was Bertrand Russell who was the most "in revolt" against psychophysical dualism, the "real aberration of seventeenth-century philosophy," which "must be annulled" (p. 235). Around the turn of the century is Freud's heroic efforts on libido theory, which, in addition to unifying all known psychologies of the time, also linked the "two realms" of mind and body (Makari, 2009, p. 120).

In the early 20th century, a new generation of heroic transcenders came on the scene. Fittingly, I start this group with Jung, who famously broke with Freud around this time. For Ponte and Schäfer's (2013), it was Jung who "had the courage" to challenge the "totalitarian materialistic environment" inaugurated by Descartes (p. 602). But this may have been a lifelong effort, for it was only in Jung's later career where we find "the great breakthrough, which put an end to the dualism of psyche and matter. . . achieved by Jung in his work on synchronicity" (von Franz, 1992, p. 159). At around the same time, Wittgenstein was being celebrated for having "fired a broadside into the Cartesian conception of the mind and sunk it once for all" (Baker & Morris, 2002, p. 161). In a similar way, other theorists regard Heidegger and his *Dasein* as providing the necessary breakthrough, which "sought interpretively to refind the unity of our Being, split asunder in the Cartesian bifurcation" (Stolorow, 2013, p. 211).

The work continues in the middle of the 20th century. For Gragg (1973), Hartshorne deserves to be recognized, for his panpsychism "repudiates metaphysical dualism in Cartesian or other forms" (p. 20), and "his anthropology rejects the. . . notion, explicitly advocated by Plato and Descartes, that man is basically a dualistic being" (p. 40). For Avens (1988), Henry Corbin shares a kinship with Swedenborg as one of the few protectors of "the third realm" (p. 382).

Gregory Bateson is also recognized for his efforts. For Graffman (2017), Bateson's work could "transcend our ancient dualisms; which Descartes in Bateson's view had made even worse with his separation of mind from body" (p. 147). Specifically, it was Bateson's "recursive epistemology" which linked the organic and inorganic, thereby "truly transcending Cartesian dualism" (p. 154). According to Small (1998), Bateson's original questioning of dualism eventually found the support of later pioneers in neuroscience. Once all this work is properly understood, "the Cartesian split. . . ceases to exist" (p. 52). But perhaps all of his followers just needed to read Bateson's (1979) own *Mind and Nature*, in which he boldly declares that dualism is heretofore "obsolete" (p. 217).

Back in the humanities, Merleau-Ponty was finishing the work that Husserl started, now wholly rejecting the "disembodied, transcendental ego," in favor of a "radical" mind-body union (Abram, 1997, p. 45). Similarly, for Temple-Hoon (2012), Merleau-Ponty "collapses the Cartesian mind/body dualism" (p. 53). Interestingly, in the same work, Merleau-Ponty also provides the foundation for "abandoning Cartesian dualism" (p. 21), even though this should not be necessary if he already collapsed it. Perhaps here it is being dimly recognized that such collapsing is an ongoing endeavor. In a related field, Gadamer finds a way "to move beyond the Cartesian Anxiety and a way out of our seduction by the dichotomy" (Smith, 1985, para. 9). Later, Gadamer gains allies. "Bernstein, Gadamer, Rorty, and others. . . are trying to release us from the grip of the Cartesian Anxiety and the dichotomy of objectivism-relativism" (para. 15). Finally, Marilyn Ferguson also "rejects Cartesian thinking" (Cee, 2013, p. 68), and Leder aims to break-up "the 'conceptual hegemony' of Cartesian dualism" (Orr, 2007, p. 103). Meanwhile, in depth psychology, "Giegerich moves out of the Cartesian either/or model," and also rescues "not the image from Cartesian banishment, but thought from its split-off position in the life world" (Temple-Hoon, 2012, pp. 10–12).

Meanwhile, the efforts continue in the sciences. Of course, Damasio is lauded, because he is critical of the Cartesian Split, both between mind and matter and between reason and emotion. He is joined by various quantum physicists, who have "attempted to bridge the division between mind and matter," and most notable for this is the work of David Bohm (Obeyesekere, 2012, p. 8). But for Capra (1983), this was more than just an attempt, for modern physics in general "shattered" the Cartesian worldview (p. 74). In biology, Maturana and Varela seek to develop theories "in a non-Cartesian way, breaking down the conceptual division between mind and world" (Colman, 2015, p. 316). Dennett (1995), perhaps inspired by science, considers himself as one of the few that have "battled Descartes' vision" (p. 3). Finally, for Berman (1981), once we discard the Western "subject/object distinction... we enter the world of sensual science, and leave Descartes behind once and for all" (p. 183). But perhaps the true solution is only in the outer edges of science, such as in panpsychism, where a "small but very significant minority of philosophers," are beginning to finally win the battle over the Cartesian view of the human-only mind (Skrbina, 2007, p. 387). Put simply, "panpsychism seeks to fuse Descartes' division by placing mind *in* matter" (Sjöstedt-H, 2018, p. 4).

Perhaps the solution is found in a field uniquely between science and the humanities, such as ecopsychology. For the name of this field alone "neatly explodes this age-old divide between mind and matter," and the inner and the outer (Fisher, 2002, p. ix). Further, "ecopsychologists reject the presumed dichotomies that underlie the modern enterprise, especially the human/nature and inner/outer splits." The task is also a noble one; it is for "healing our dualism by returning soul to nature and nature to soul" (pp. 9–10). For Oelschlager, Abram's ecopsychology "magically subverts the dichotomies of culture and nature, body and mind" (as cited in Abram, 1997, p. iii).

I conclude this section with some transcenders from some unlikely sources, far outside of the academy. Evidently, Pentacostal-Charismatic Christians also reject "a Cartesian dualism that separates body from spirit" (Poloma, 2003, p. 22). Through their practices, they demonstrate freedom from the dominant Cartesian split, holistically integrating "soul, spirit, mind and body" (pp. 87–88). Also, for all these challenges requiring bold heroes, the solution may in fact be found in everyday experience. Michael Ventura argues that black culture and black music has healed and transcended the Cartesian split (as cited in Dyson, 2001, p. 317). Van Dijk and Hummels (2017) aim to "overcome two, strongly related, lingering 'Cartesian' splits," noting that "the hammer and the blind man's cane have famously been used to argue against a strict separation" (p. 48).

Tragic transcenders

Considering all the great thinkers who have battled and rejected the Cartesian Split, over centuries, it would seem assured that the work would be complete by now. And yet, judging from the publication dates of the latter sources, the battle rages on, perhaps even increasing in intensity. Fortunately, the Cartesian Split complex can properly account for this curiosity. It actually turns out to be very common, although not in the abstracts, for a heroic transcender to also be portrayed as a failure. The hero fights the good fight, but tragically remains embedded within the all-powerful Cartesian legacy, in spite of all their valiant efforts. This is of course required considering the theme of the (currently) Dominant Paradigm. It may also serve the purpose of telling a better story, for if every previous hero has failed, the next hero is to be celebrated even more.

Many of these examples include some of the luminaries noted above. The first of those who fought but failed is Kant, who, as a "courageous pioneer," tried to "reconcile the widely divergent streams that traced their source to Descartes." But he failed, because "he never discarded the fatal Cartesian hypothesis" that ideas are not naturally related to objects (Temple, 1934, pp. 70–71). Husserl, despite all of his work, "was unable to drop the transcendental, idealist aspirations of his early philosophy," in which the self was separable from the body" (Abram, 1997, p. 45). Whitehead's objective realism was "radically different," but in the end, it is still a realism, and thus a distinction between sensations and that which causes the sensations. Thus "the assailant of dualism becomes its defender and elaborator" (Lovejoy, 1955, pp. 193–194). Similarly, Polanyi is "caught in the Cartesianism he rejects," unable to link the visceral and the cerebral (Berman, 1981, p. 155). According to Bernstein (as cited in J. K. Smith, 1985), although Gadamer found a way out of our seduction, ultimately, he does not succeed (para. 11). In feminist studies, academic critiques of Cartesianism do so in a way that regrettably preserves it. "Although Cartesian Man has been officially declared dead, like Freddy Kruger he just keeps popping up again—particularly in academia!" (Bordo, 1999, p. 19).

The situation is no better in depth psychology. Freud perhaps gets most of the tragic laments here, in spite of his libido theory, previously celebrated for linking mind and body. And yet, it required the intersubjectivists, "critics of Freud's Cartesianism," to finally recognize the "thirdness" between subjects (Benjamin, 2004, para. 4). Also, Atwood et al (2011) spent 35 years of their careers "devoted to liberating psychoanalytic theory and practice from various forms of Cartesian, isolated-mind thinking en route to a post-Cartesian psychoanalytic perspective" (p. 263). Similarly, Freud's topography is a "neo-Cartesian id-ego-superego model" (Obeyesekere, 2012, p. 8). But perhaps all of this commentary is unnecessary, for "Freud, as is well known, adhered religiously to the Cartesian paradigm" (Berman, 1981, p. 172).

However, those who followed in Freud's footsteps unfortunately followed the same tragic path. Reich and Jung challenge Cartesianism, but cannot quite replace it (Berman, 1981, p. 156). And Jung's synchronicity, earlier lauded as the final breakthrough, only "seems such a direct challenge to the Cartesian split." But this solution "remains symptomatic of a dualistic world-view" (Colman, 2015, p. 316). Still, the effort is noted, being described by another author as a "desperate effort to bridge an unbridgeable chasm" (p. 320). Perhaps this was due to the fact that Jung was implying the very same dualism he was trying to overcome (p. 317). The tragic pattern continues in neo-Jungians. "Giegerich's thoughts extend from Cartesian, specifically Hegelian, philosophy and remain Cartesian in the elevation of the thinking mind over the world" (Temple-Hoon, 2012, p. 74). Further, "like Jung, Hillman laments but does not dispense with the Cartesian dualistic assumptions" (p. 69).

Battles were fought and lost in the sciences as well. Although Faraday was one of the first "go beyond" the mechanical philosophy, it "still held its position" (Capra, 1983, p. 70). And although modern physics "shattered" the Cartesian worldview, one of its greatest proponents was unable to himself break free. "Einstein's philosophy was essentially Cartesian." Also, "it seems that Einstein, somehow, could not bring himself to go beyond Descartes" (p. 82). The other side of modern physics did not fare any better. "Despite the discoveries of quantum physics, the mind-body split in Western medicine prevails" (Lipton, 2008, p. 95).

To sum up, according to Smith (2011), "while science claims to have long ago rejected a Cartesian view of the world, in fact the influence of this philosopher is still immense" (para. 3). Further "science has a sort of schizoid relationship with Descartes, in some respects firmly rejecting his views, but in other respects still clinging to them" (para. 34). Even Daniel Dennett, "a hard core materialist if ever there were one" (para. 37), is yet "still in the thrall of Cartesianism" (para. 40).

Various other examples in other fields can be found. For one, behaviorists try to transcend, but "remain caught in the absurdity of the Cartesian split" (Small, 1998, p. 52). Although physical education pioneer Margaret Whitehead intends to challenge the Cartesian paradigm, her "referral to the body as an 'instrument of expression,' . . . perpetuates the Cartesian divide in such dualistic language" (R. J. Lloyd, 2011, p. 76). Brady (1981) notes Comfort's critique of the "Cartesian Observer," but this critique unfortunately creates more problems than it solves. "Mr. Comfort's technique is more Cartesian than he admits" (p. 211). Feminism also falls away defeated, for "this tension surrounding representation actually sustains the Cartesian mind/body dualism that it ostensibly criticizes" (Bray & Colebrook, 1998, p. 35). Finally, the entirety of the postmodern movement, in spite of all of its efforts to emancipate itself from it, is still a "direct descendent of the Cartesian legacy" (Thomas, 1996, p. 1).

For Walker Percy, from which comes "the dread chasm," the problem takes on new dimensions. Percy (1990) argues that the split is so dominant, that it is felt by each and every one of us, whenever we even think of the opposed terms, "the 'mental' and the 'physical.'" But the magnitude of the problem is matched only by its invisibility. We suspect that there is a problem between these two terms, but do not acknowledge it. If we are honest, "are we not admitting that we are still hung up on the horns of the ancient dualism of Descartes, however much we wish to believe we had gotten past it?" (p. 3). For these reasons, he gives the Cartesian Split a new, dramatic name, also the title of the article. It is "The Fateful Rift: The San Andreas Fault in the Modern Mind." From this perspective, not only have all the great battles been lost, but now the enemy looms larger, and worse, completely unseen. Thus, it is easy to find a recent internet article which does not even acknowledge the widespread problem. "Most people realize that the mind and body are connected. . . 'A healthy mind in a healthy body,'" so *say* "psychologists and physicians alike" (James, 2019, para. 1). The Cartesian Split is truly nowhere. And so, we appear to be at a dead end. With every attack, the Cartesian Split gets stronger, more pervasive, and now, more invisible.

This dilemma sets up another fractal level of meaning when compared to the theme of the Old versus New. In short, as the Old grows stronger, the efficacy of the New must wane. Recall that all the geniuses of modern physics, as well as the entirety of the postmodern movement, could not break free of the Old. This presents a rather uncomfortable doubt. Essentially, if Einstein was not New enough, we may well be running out of the New, emptying the future. This may be why, for Percy (1990), the solution to the "Fateful Rift" is not new, but to revisit the 19th century, to study C. S. Peirce. And this may not even go far enough back for Damasio, whose follow-up to *Descartes' Error* is titled *Looking for Spinoza*. Perhaps what is Old is yet New again.

There is yet another level to all this. If we were to go all the way back to Descartes himself, we also find the unusual critique that he himself was a prime heroic rejecter and transcender. After all, what other than a heroic "father" could single-handedly displace Aristotle and scholasticism, which was taught for thousand years in all the best schools? Who else could end the primitive superstition of the Middle Ages, and single-handedly usher in the modern period? Notably, Descartes seems to be the only heroic transcender in this tradition not also a tragic transcender.

As such, what is really remarkable about these critiques is that there is a certain longing for a return to the time *before* Descartes. This was certainly the sentiment of the Pope and is echoed in other sources. For Berman (1981), after Descartes "took his stand against Scholasticism," rejecting the best of Europe's achievements (pp. 31–32), what replaced it was alienation and disenchantment. "Medieval man" no longer had a "purposeful position in the universe." And even though they dealt with plague and natural disaster, their environment was somehow "psychologically reassuring" (pp. 51–52). "Original participation" in the cosmos was "finally ousted" (p. 73). The "organic" universe of the Middle Ages is lost, thanks to the Cartesian turn, and its "rejection" of all values associated with that world (Bordo, 1987, pp. 7–9). The Cartesian machine model violated "the old kindly fellowship of living things" (Cottingham, 1998, p. 225).

Thus, with a supreme but unnoticed sense of irony, we must now reject and transcend that which previously rejected and transcended, in favor of that which was rejected and transcended. To follow these leads would seem to take us on an infinite time-loop of perpetual rejecting and transcending. It is no wonder that all who have ever taken on this charge have tragically failed, and the dread chasm, while invisible, looms larger than ever before.

Charged images

The final theme worth noting is the highly charged language and somewhat disturbing tone that often accompanies the Split. Some of the quotes I have already provided demonstrate this, but three works in particular offer noteworthy examples. Expanding on an earlier example, Lock (2002) paints a rather disturbing image of doctors pronouncing patients brain-dead, in order to harvest their organs, while they are still alive. What is unusual is, again, the choice of words. The Cartesian Split "allows" them to do this, almost as if it allows a somewhat malicious part of the doctor's intentions to prevail, against their better wishes. For Mills (2006), a figure in the field has regrettably committed the error of maintaining "the deadly Cartesian split of objective onlooker." Finally, summarizing several of the above themes, Mortimore (2013) states that ecological ways of living have been "disregarded, discarded, and destroyed" on account of the split, whose "hegemonic layers of control have served to bind the fate of the Earth's eco-systems."

Other sources also demonstrate images of a traumatic nature and are often accompanied with terms of severe psychopathology. For example, there is an online video of a popular science researcher, Edward Frenkel, titled "Cartesianism as the Effect of our Collective Childhood Trauma" (scienceandnonduality, 2015). Interestingly, having watched the video, the speaker says almost nothing about Descartes, so something else must have motivated the choice of title. For Smith (1985), if we cannot "exorcise this Cartesian Anxiety," then "we cannot escape the forces of darkness that envelop us with madness, with intellectual and moral chaos" (para. 5). For Temple-Hoon (2012), it was "Cartesian philosophy that sacrificed the earth and the body" (p. 21), and "the ego of Cartesian philosophy and modem science ravaged life and banished its mystery to an imaginal realm" (p. 70). Bateson (2000) takes up a fatalistic stance, for with Cartesian dualism, "it is doubtful whether a species having both an advanced technology and this strange way of looking at its world can endure" (p. 337).

There are also images of physical violence. According to Percy (as cited in Busch & Lawler, 2009), the Cartesian self is a "self ripped from self and man pasted back together as mythical monster, half angel, half beast, but no man (p. 103). But according to some countercultural critics, there is no pasting back together, but only a "Cartesian severed head and divided self" that remains (Gilman, 1993, p. 243). However, these are not just metaphors. It has been suggested that such theories of mind-body division can lead to a physical enactment, including a mother actually decapitating her children. Unaware of the influence of unconscious theories, "our civilization. . . has achieved a systemic mind-body split that is in fact killing our children" (Gallop, 1988, pp. 1–2).

Further, for Cody (2016), "The ontology of the moderns, Descartes' in particular," can be considered "the cannibalism of the individual's own flesh" (p. 6). Also, quoting another source, "the American individual has been 'afflicted with a particularly virulent strain of this Cartesian malady'" (p. 10). The split also justifies racism through "robbing them of a soul" (p. 36). Colonialism, the American Civil War and both World Wars are all caused by Cartesian Dualism (p. 45).

Others join in on Whitehead's evaluation of dualism as a "disastrous" moment. Temple (1934) judges it to be the "most disastrous moment in the history of Europe," leading to, with no doubt, "many of our worst troubles, not only in philosophy but also in politics and economics" (p. 57). Similarly, for Koestler (1964), "modern philosophy starts with what one might call the Cartesian Catastrophe," which was "the splitting up of the world into the realms of matter and mind, and the identification of 'mind' with conscious thinking" (p. 148). Finally, on a popular Catholic podcast, the host recalls a speech from a college professor, who always used to refer to the *cogito* as "the rape and pillage of the universe," and "the destruction of the universe by this one phrase" (Nepil, n.d.).

First evaluation

As can be seen, there is a very wide array of related but disparate themes attached to the idea of the Cartesian Split. From this perspective, the authors of these works can be forgiven for never defining what they mean by that exact phrase, because it cannot be precisely defined. The only common definition that could be gleaned from this survey is that the Cartesian Split is a very bad thing, and has been so in the Western world for centuries. This situation is not unlike that of our hypothetical Ash, whose father complex does not always hang together logically, but at least we can be sure it is beheld as negative.

However, there is one way to gain a higher perspective of the elements of this overall *complex* of ideas, and that is a graphical form. To do this, I wrote down each theme onto a blank sheet, in the form of multiple text boxes, using different font sizes to correlate with the number of times each theme was present in the original 34 specimens. I then linked the boxes to

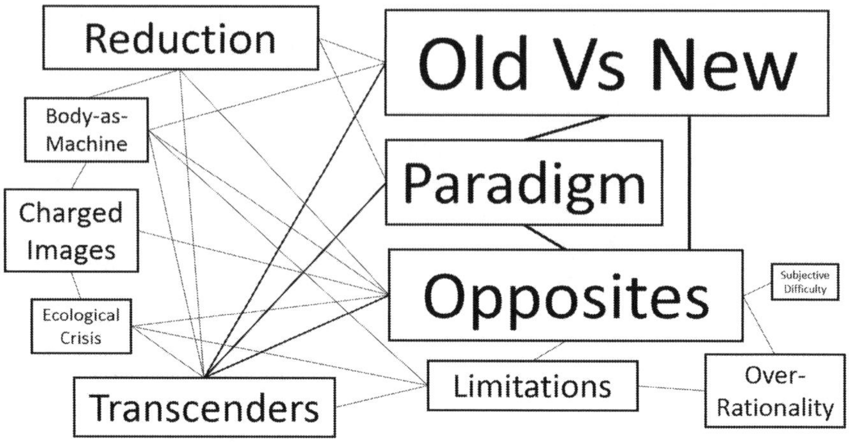

Figure 2.1 Thematic map of the survey of abstracts.

show how some themes appear to be expressed more prominently along with certain others. Stronger relationships are denoted by thicker lines. Although some of my decisions for this may have been arbitrary, I hope this will allow for a better conception of the different themes, their strength of expression, and how they relate to each other.

At this point, it would be fair to wonder what relationship, if at all, this complex of ideas has toward its original subject matter, the philosophical dualism of Descartes. Ostensibly, all of these highly detailed discussions on different topics in different fields all originated from one man's personal musings on the nature of mind and body, almost 400 years ago. I have already argued that there really is no relationship, or at least the linkage is so strained it almost inconsequential. But let us see if comparing these themes to the original subject matter allows any further understanding of the structure of this complex. In other words, if all of this really comes from a distinction between "mind" and "body," then where would these terms fall onto this map?

First, "mind" would seem to locate in the lower right corner, near the theme of Over-rationality and Subjective Difficulty. Conversely, "body" gravitates toward the upper left, near Body-as-Machine and Mechanistic Reduction. But this itself is quite curious. Supposedly, the split is a radical split, the "abyssal separation" of Damasio, or the "dread chasm" of Percy. Further, it is traditionally known that Descartes favored only one side of the split, the mind. If the split is as truly as radical as is claimed, then "body" should not even be part of this discussion. But there it is, looming large, particularly as the infamous "Machine" metaphor, that which has dominated Western medicine for centuries, while also manifesting as the Ecological Crisis. Further, it the split is as radical as believed, why are these two regions so closely linked? In some of my sources, an over-emphasis on reason somehow leads directly to mechanism and ecological destruction. Perhaps the split is not so radical as is commonly believed. I believe this is an especially important irony, a critical tension that is inherent to the core meaning of the Cartesian Split complex, and I will be further drawing out and elaborating on this throughout the remainder of this book.

References

Abram, D. (1997). *The spell of the sensuous: Perception and language in a more-than-human world*. New York, NY: Vintage Books.

Abram, D. (2002). Foreword. In *Radical ecopsychology: Psychology in the service of life* (pp. ix–xi). Albany: State University of New York Press.

Ariew, R. (1992). Descartes and scholasticism: The intellectual background to Descartes' thought. In J. Cottingham (Ed.), *The Cambridge companion to Descartes* (pp. 58–90). Cambridge, UK: Cambridge University Press.

Atwood, G. E., Stolorow, R. D., & Orange, D. M. (2011). The madness and genius of post-Cartesian philosophy: A distant mirror. *The Psychoanalytic Review*, *98*(3), 263–285. doi: 10.1521/prev.2011.98.3.263

Avens, R. (1988). The subtle realm: Corbin, Sufism and Swedenborg. In R. Larsen (Ed.), *Emanuel Swedenborg: A continuing vision: A pictorial biography & anthology of essays & poetry* (pp. 382–391). New York, NY: Swedenborg Foundation.

Baker, G. P., & Morris, K. J. (2002). *Descartes' dualism*. London, UK: Routledge.

Balzac, S. (2008). *Tips for parents: Cartesian splits and Chinese splits*. Davidson Institute for Talent Development. Retrieved from: https://www.davidsongifted.org/Search-Database/entry/A10519

Bankart, C. P. (2006). Treating anger with wisdom and compassion: A buddhist approach. In E. L. Feindler (Ed.), *Anger related disorders: A practitioner's guide to comparative treatments* (2006–05844-011; pp. 231–255). Springer; psyh. Retrieved from: http://pgi.idm.oclc.org/login?url=http://search.ebscohost.com/login.aspx?direct=true&db=psyh&AN=2006-05844-011&site=ehost-live&scope=site

Barron, R. (2015, June 9). Bruce Jenner, the "shadow council," and St. Irenaeus. *Word on fire*. Retrieved from: https://www.wordonfire.org/resources/article/bruce-jenner-the-shadow-council-and-st-irenaeus/4785/

Bateson, G. (1979). *Mind and nature: A necessary unity* (1st ed.). New York, NY: Dutton.

Bateson, G. (2000). *Steps to an ecology of mind*. Chicago, IL: University of Chicago Press.

Bendelow, G. (2006). Pain, suffering and risk. *Health, Risk and Society*, *8*(1), 59–70.

Benjamin, J. (2004). Beyond doer and done to: An intersubjective view of thirdness. *Psychoanalytic Quarterly*, *73*, 5–46.

Berman, M. (1981). *The reenchantment of the world*. Ithaca, NY: Cornell University Press.

Bordo, S. (1987). *The flight to objectivity: Essays on Cartesianism and culture.* Albany: State University of New York Press.

Bordo, S. (1999). Introduction. In S. Bordo (Ed.), *Feminist interpretations of René Descartes* (pp. 1–25). University Park: Pennsylvania State University Press.

Brady, R. (1977). Goethe's natural science: Some non-Cartesian meditations. *Toward a Man-Centered Science, 1*, 137–165.

Brady, R. (1981). Minds, models and Cartesian observers: A note on conceptual problems. *Journal of Social and Biological Structures, 4*(3), 277–286.

Bray, A., & Colebrook, C. (1998). The haunted flesh: Corporeal feminism and the politics of (dis)embodiment. *Signs: Journal of Women in Culture and Society, 24*(1), 35–67. doi: 10.1086/495317

Brencick, J. M. (1997). *Universality and singularity: A philosophy of nursing* (UMI 9804624) [Doctoral dissertation]. ProQuest Dissertations and Theses.

Bright, B. (2015). *Culture collapse disorder: Ecopsychopathy, exile, and the end of home* (UMI 3684129) [Doctoral dissertation]. ProQuest Dissertations and Theses.

Busch, E. K., & Lawler, P. A. (2009). *Democracy reconsidered.* Lanham, MD: Lexington Books.

Capra, F. (1983). *The turning point: Science, society, and the rising culture.* New York, NY: Bantam Books.

Cee, V. (2013). The end(s) of advocacy: Responding to our own mandates instead of creating new leadership. *Action, Criticism, and Theory for Music Education, 12*(1), 64–81.

Cody, T. (2016). Lillian Smith, Richard Wright, and Walker Percy's ontological vision: Gnosticism, Cartesian dualism, and the split of the Southern self. *Theses and Dissertations.* Retrieved from: https://scholarcommons.sc.edu/etd/3461

Colman, W. (2015). Bounded in a nutshell and a king of infinite space: The embodied self and its intentional world: The embodied self and its intentional world. *Journal of Analytical Psychology, 60*(3), 316–335. doi: 10.1111/1468-5922.12152

Conway, M., & Pratt, N. (2019, February 10). *Art in general.* Retrieved from: http://www.artingeneral.org/exhibitions/237

Cortesi, T. (2013). *"Traitorous bodies": Cartesian dualism in romance novels by Susan Johnson and E.L. James* [Master's Thesis]. Texas State University.

Cottingham, J. (1998). Descartes' treatment of animals. In J. Cottingham (Ed.), *Descartes* (pp. 225–233). Oxford, UK: Oxford University Press.

Cushman, P. (2011). So who's asking? Politics, hermeneutics, and individuality. In R. Frie & W. J. Coburn (Eds.), *Persons in context: The challenge of individuality in theory and practice* (2010–09131-002; Vol. 32, pp. 21–40). Routledge/Taylor & Francis; PsycINFO. Retrieved from: http://pgi.idm.oclc.org/login?url=http://search.ebscohost.com/login.aspx?direct=true&db=psyh&AN=2010-09131-002&site=ehost-live&scope=site

de Quincey, C. (2008). Reality bubbles: Can we know anything about the physical world? *Journal of Consciousness Studies, 15*(8), 94–101.

Dennett, D. (1995). Review of Damasio, Descartes' error. In *Times Literary Supplement* (pp. 3–4). Times Newspapers Ltd. Retrieved from: https://ase.tufts.edu/cogstud/dennett/papers/damasio.htm

Dyson, M. E. (2001). When you divide body and soul, problems multiply: The black church and sex. In R. P. Byrd & B. Guy-Sheftall (Eds.), *Traps: African*

American Men on Gender and Sexuality (pp. 308–326). Bloomington: Indiana University Press.

Fenwick, S. M. (1998). *The dreaming earth: Foundations for a process-oriented approach to ecopsychology*. (UMI 9910825) [Doctoral dissertation]. ProQuest Dissertations and Theses.

Fisanick, C. L. (2003). *The embodied pedagogue: Teaching and writing with the body* (UMI 3099577) [Doctoral dissertation]. ProQuest Dissertations and Theses.

Fisher, A. (2002). *Radical ecopsychology: Psychology in the service of life*. Albany: State University of New York Press.

Forsman, J. (2015). *Did Descartes kick dogs? Some words on the Cartesian conception of animals*. Retrieved from: https://www.academia.edu/31979299/Did_Descartes_kick_dogs_Some_words_on_the_Cartesian_conception_of_animals

Gallop, J. (1988). *Thinking through the body*. New York, NY: Columbia University Press.

Gaukroger, S. (1998). *Descartes: An intellectual biography*. Oxford, UK: Clarendon Press.

Gilman, S. L. (1993). *Hysteria beyond Freud*. Berkeley: University of California Press.

Goebel, E. (2014). The one-way road of aging: On Jean Améry's essay über das altern. *The Germanic Review*, *89*(2), 202–211. eoah.

Goodrich, A. (2004). Scaling culture: Rock climbing and the embodied nature of spatial knowledge. *Anthropology Southern Africa*, *27*(1–2), 27–34. eoah.

Graffman, E. (2017). On Gregory Bateson's epistemology, his definition of mind, and its solution to the Cartesian dualism or mind-body problem. *Rocznik Naukowy Kujawsko-Pomorskiej Szkoły Wyższej w Bydgoszczy. Transdyscyplinarne Studia o Kulturze (i) Edukacji*, *12*, 146–157.

Gragg, A. (1973). *Charles Hartshorne. Word Books*. Retrieved from: http://www.religion-online.org/book/charles-hartshorne/

Güzeldere, G., & Franchi, S. (1995). Mindless mechanisms, mindful constructions. *Stanford Electronic Humanities Review*, *4*(2). Retrieved from: http://web.stanford.edu/group/SHR/4-2/text/introduction.html#note3

Hannah, B. (1976). *Jung, his life and work: A biographical memoir*. New York, NY: Putnam.

Hoeppe, G. (2015). Representing representation. *Science, Technology and Human Values*, *40*(6), 1077–1092. eoah.

Hollomon, D. (2000). *The "I" of the therapist: Eastern mindfulness and the skillful use of self in psychotherapy*. (UMI 9976891) [Doctoral dissertation]. ProQuest Dissertations and Theses.

Iltis, C. (1973). The decline of Cartesianism in mechanics: The Leibnizian-Cartesian debates. *Isis*, *64*(3), 356–373.

Isaacs, W. N. (2001). Toward an action theory of dialogue. *International Journal of Public Administration*, *24*(7–8), 709–748. eoah.

James, G. (2019, July 5). *Neuroscience says your body and mind get stronger when you focus on this one thing*. Inc.Com. Retrieved from: https://www.inc.com/geoffrey-james/neuroscience-says-your-body-mind-get-stronger-when-you-focus-on-this-one-thingdraft-1562273865.html

Jolley, N. (1992). The reception of Descartes' philosophy. In J. Cottingham (Ed.), *The Cambridge companion to Descartes* (pp. 393–423). Cambridge, UK: Cambridge University Press.

Kavanagh, A. M., & Broom, D. H. (1998). Embodied risk: My body, myself? *Social Science and Medicine*, *46*(3), 437–444. doi: 10.1016/S0277-9536(97)00188-3

Kellogg, C. (2013). *Road back to recovery: Hermeneutic phenomenological inquiry into psychotropic medication management*. doi: 10.1037/e621642013-001

Kelso, C. (2015, February 10). Reuniting the apparent mind/body split. *The Deepest Peace*. Retrieved from: https://thedeepestpeace.com/2015/02/10/reuniting-the-apparent-mindbody-split/#more-413

Koestler, A. (1964). *The act of creation*. London, UK: Hutchinson & Co.

Koopman, K. (2019, February 10). *Cartesian split (excerpt)*. Retrieved from: https://soundcloud.com/athrynoopman/cartesian-split-excerpt

Kureethadam, J. I. (2017). *The philosophical roots of the ecological crisis: Descartes and the modern worldview*. Newcastle upon Tyne, UK: Cambridge Scholars Publishing.

Lapointe, F. H. (1976). The existence of alter egos: Jean-Paul Sartre and Maurice Merleau-Ponty. *Journal of Phenomenological Psychology*, *6*(2), 209–216. psyh. doi: 10.1163/156916276X00089

Lee, K. (2013). *Reading Descartes otherwise: Blind, mad, dreamy, and bad*. New York, NY: Fordham University Press.

Lerner, R. (1999). Review of the book Synthesizing nature-nurture: Prenatal roots of instinctive behavior by G. Gottlieb. *International Journal of Behavioral Development*, *23*(1), 265–272. eoah.

Lipton, B. H. (2008). *The biology of belief: Unleashing the power of consciousness, matter & miracles*. Carlsbad, CA: Hay House.

Lloyd, G. (1993). *The man of reason: Male and "female" in western philosophy* (2nd ed.). London, UK: Routledge.

Lloyd, R. J. (2011). Awakening movement consciousness in the physical landscapes of literacy: Leaving, reading and being moved by one's trace. *Phenomenology & Practice*, *5*(2), 73–92. doi: 10.29173/pandpr19846

Lock, M. (2002). Inventing a new death and making it believable. *Anthropology and Medicine*, *9*(2), 97–115. eoah.

Lokhorst, G. (2016). Descartes and the pineal gland. In E. N. Zalta (Ed.), *The Stanford encyclopedia of philosophy*. Retrieved from: http://plato.stanford.edu/archives/sum2016/entries/pineal-gland/

Lovejoy, A. O. (1955). *The revolt against dualism: An inquiry concerning the existence of ideas*. LaSalle, IL: Open Court Publishing.

Maddock, M., & Humphries, M. (2010). Perspectives on the social implications of developments in quantum physics with a focus on reuniting the Cartesian split. *Organization, Identity and Locality (OIL) VI: Critical Studies of Management and Organizing in Aotearoa/New Zealand*, 52–57. Retrieved from: http://citeseerx.ist.psu.edu/viewdoc/download?doi=10.1.1.456.9464&rep=rep1&type=pdf#page=52

Maguire, R. (1997). "Proofs of God's existence:" Walker Percy, Jacques Maritain, and the problem of the symbol in the moviegoer. *Logos: A Journal of Catholic Thought and Culture*, *1*(3), 69–79. doi: 10.1353/log.1997.0018

Makari, G. (2009). *Revolution in mind: The creation of psychoanalysis*. New York, NY: Harper Perennial.

Marshall, P. J. (2015). Neuroscience, embodiment, and development. In W. F. Overton, P. C. M. Molenaar, & R. M. Lerner (Eds.), *Handbook of child psychology and developmental science, Vol. 1: Theory and method*

(7th ed.) (2015–15498-007; pp. 244–283). Wiley; psyh. Retrieved from: http://pgi.idm.oclc.org/login?url=http://search.ebscohost.com/login.aspx?direct=true&db=psyh&AN=2015-15498-007&site=ehost-live&scope=site

Metzger, J. G. (1987). *Narration as a construct for understanding third-culture building: Exploring missionaries' success and effectiveness as cosmological change agents* (UMI DP22421) [Doctoral dissertation]. ProQuest Dissertations and Theses.

Mills, B. (2006). Jung and the African diaspora. *Western Journal of Black Studies*, *30*(2), 84–88.

Mkhatshwa, E. (2010). Authorial intention and agency in Luke's Acts. *Outeursintensie En Handelingsrol in Lukas Se Handelinge*, *31*(1), 99–122.

Mortimore, L. (2013). *Embodied ways of knowing: Women's eco-activism* (Accession or Order No. NS28393) [Doctoral dissertation]. ProQuest Dissertations and Theses.

Nepil, J. (n.d.). *The Cartesian demiurge*. Retrieved February 17, 2019, from https://catholicstuffpodcast.com/podcast/2014/12/01/the-cartesian-demiurge.html

Obeyesekere, G. (2012). *The awakened ones: Phenomenology of visionary experience*. New York, NY: Columbia University Press.

Orning, S. E. S. (2012). *Fleshly embodiments: Early modern monsters, Victorian freaks, and twentieth-century affective spectatorship* (UMI 3521806) [Doctoral dissertation]. ProQuest Dissertations and Theses.

Orr, D. (2007). *Feminist politics: Identity, difference, and agency*. Lanham, MD: Rowman & Littlefield.

Overton, W. F. (2013). A new paradigm for developmental science: Relationism and relational-developmental systems. *Applied Developmental Science*, *17*(2), 94–107. eoah.

Paul II, P. J. & Messori, V. (1994). *Crossing the threshold of hope. Knopf.* Retrieved from: http://search.ebscohost.com/login.aspx?direct=true&scope=site&db=nlebk&db=nlabk&AN=718803

Percy, W. (1990). The fateful rift: The San Andreas fault in the modern mind. *Design for Arts in Education*, *91*(3), 2–7, 51–53.

Pether, P. (1999). On foreign ground: Grand narratives, situated specificities, and the praxis of critical theory and law. *Law and Critique*, *10*(3), 211–236. eoah.

Poloma, M. M. (2003). *Main street mystics: The Toronto blessing and reviving pentecostalism*. Walnut Creek, CA: Altamira.

Pope, C. (2011, April 5). On the Cartesian anxiety of our times and what faith can offer. *Community in Mission*. Retrieved from: http://blog.adw.org/2011/04/on-the-cartesian-anxiety-of-our-times-and-what-faith-can-offer/

Potter, B. (2011). The hallowed in the hollow: Aesthetic elements of the sublime in the Cartesian unworld. *Avello Publishing Journal*, *1*(1), 23–42.

Reid-Pharr, R. (1999). *Conjugal union: The body, the house, and the black American*. New York, NY: Oxford University Press.

Rosado, C. (2008). Context determines content: Quantum physics as a framework for "wholeness" in urban transformation. *Urban Studies*, *45*(10), 2075–2097.

Schwyzer, H. (1997). Subjectivity in Descartes and Kant. *The Philosophical Quarterly*, *47*(188), 342–357.

Scienceandnonduality. (2015, December 16). *Cartesianism as the effect of our collective childhood trauma, Edward Frenkel*. Retrieved from: https://www.youtube.com/watch?v=t_iE04ggR9w

Seidl, C. (2013, January 10). *The Cartesian paradigm.* Retrieved from: http://www.carlaseidl.com/2013/the-cartesian-paradigm/

Shapiro, Y. (2015). Dynamical systems therapy (DST): Theory and practical applications. *Psychoanalytic Dialogues*, *25*(1), 83–107. eoah.

Sheldrake, R. (2012). *Science set free: 10 paths to new discovery.* New York, NY: Deepak Chopra Books.

Silverstein, C. M. (2003). *Looking back to the future in nursing science development from 1952–2002: A historical perspective* (UMI 3091294) [Doctoral dissertation]. ProQuest Dissertations and Theses.

Sjöstedt-H, P. (2018). Panpsychism: Ubiquitous sentience. *High Existence, 1.*

Skrbina, D. (2007). Beyond Descartes: Panpsychism revisited. *Axiomathes*, *16*(4), 387–423. doi: 10.1007/s10516-005-8708-3

Small, C. (1998). *Musicking: The meanings of performing and listening.* Middletown, CT: Wesleyan University Press.

Smith, A. P. (2011, October). Do we need an absolute? *Do We Need an Absolute?* Retrieved from: http://www.integralworld.net/smith35.html

Smith, J. K. (1985). Review of Bernstein: Beyond objectivism and relativism. *Phenomenology + Pedagogy*, *3*(1), 60–64.

Smith, M. B. (2015). William James. In J. D. Wright (Ed.), *International encyclopedia of the social & behavioral sciences* (2nd ed., pp. 786–790). Elsevier.

Snyder, G. (2001). *The practice of the wild: Essays.* New York, NY: North Point Press.

Sorell, T. (2005). *Descartes reinvented.* Cambridge, UK: Cambridge University Press.

Spuybroek, L. (1999). The Cartesian split. *ANY: Architecture New York*, *24*, 13–13. JSTOR.

Steelman, T. (2018, February 11). *Cartesian self vs. Ecological self.* Medium. Retrieved from: https://medium.com/@taylor.steelman.ot/what-is-the-most-dangerous-thing-in-existence-bb55294391c6

Stern, K. (1999). Descartes. In S. Bordo (Ed.), *Feminist interpretations of René Descartes* (pp. 29–47). University Park, PA: Pennsylvania State University Press.

Stolorow, R. D. (2013). Heidegger and post-Cartesian psychoanalysis: My personal, psychoanalytic, and philosophical sojourn. *Humanistic Psychologist*, *41*(3), 209–218. doi: 10.1080/08873267.2012.724266

Storm, S. (2015). *An elegy on species obituaries* (UMI 10001004) [Master's Thesis]. ProQuest Dissertations and Theses.

Temple, W. (1934). *Nature, man and God.* Edinburgh, UK: R. & R. Clark, Limited.

Temple-Hoon, J. (2012). *Returning to the labyrinth: The sacrificial body in Cartesian philosophy, phenomenology, and the myth of Ariadne and Theseus* (UMI 3065325) [Doctoral dissertation].

Thayer, L. L. (2009). *The adoption of shamanic healing into the biomedical health care system in the United States.* (UMI AAI3359161) [Doctoral dissertation]. ProQuest Information and Learning.

Thayer, V. T. (1919). A comparison of Bergson and Spinoza: With reference to their conceptions of reality and knowledge. *The Monist*, *29*(1), 96–105. JSTOR.

Thomas, C. C. S. (1996). *The allure of determinacy: Truth and Cartesian certainty* (UMI 9625960) [Doctoral dissertation]. ProQuest Dissertations and Theses.

Tomos, Y. (2013). *The significance of anime as a novel animation form, referencing selected works by Hayao Miyazaki, Satoshi Kon and Mamoru Oshii* [Doctoral dissertation]. Aberystwth University.

Valadas Ponte, D., & Schäfer, L. (2013). Carl Gustav Jung, quantum physics and the spiritual mind: A mystical vision of the twenty-first century. *Behavioral Sciences*, *3*(4), 601–618. doi: 10.3390/bs3040601

van Dijk, J., & Hummels, C. (2017). Designing for embodied being-in-the-world: Two cases, seven principles and one framework. *Proceedings of the Tenth International Conference on Tangible, Embedded, and Embodied Interaction - TEI'*, *17*, 47–56. doi: 10.1145/3024969.3025007

Vertinsky, P. (2001). A militant madonna: Charlotte Perkins Gilman—Feminism and physical culture. *The International Journal of the History of Sport*, *18*(1), 55–72. eoah.

Voltaire, F.-M. (1901). *The works of Voltaire, a contemporary version* (W. F. Fleming, Trans.). Retrieved from: http://archive.org/details/worksofvoltairec12volt

von Franz, M.-L. (1992). *Psyche and matter.* Boston, MA and London, UK: Shambhala.

Washburn, T. (2012). *Healing the Cartesian split: Understanding and renewing pathos in academic writing* [Master's Thesis]. Retrieved from: http://scholarsarchive.byu.edu/etd/3671

Watson, R. A. (1998). *The breakdown of Cartesian metaphysics.* Indianapolis, IN: Hackett.

Whitehead, A. N. (1938). *Modes of thought.* New York, NY: The Macmillan Company.

Whitehead, A. N. (1979). *Process and reality: An essay in cosmology* (D. R. Griffin & D. W. Sherburne, Eds.). New York, NY: Free Press.

Wilde, S. (2013). *Care in education: Teaching with understanding and compassion.* New York, NY: Routledge.

Chapter 3

The depth sessions

The initial sessions are over, the primary elements of the complex are established, and now Ash is committed to going deeper into therapy. After having captured the initial associations, and further amplifications, I will then inquire for additional, focused works. I might say to Ash, "I am very curious about this history with your Father. I want you to go home and focus on this one particular memory, and write in your journal about this one topic only." It is necessary to concentrate fully on the images that come up, what they really mean, and why they are so important right now, in the present moment, after all these years. The equivalent to this for this study would be a summary of academic works that are dedicated almost entirely to the subject of widespread, problematic Cartesian influence. These are different from most of the works cited above, in which the subject is usually invoked only to advance other arguments.

The great revolt

As documented above, the theme of the Heroic Transcender comes from a long list of sources, but there is one work in particular that almost embodies the entire theme by itself. This is a book titled *The Revolt Against Dualism*, by Arthur O. Lovejoy, commonly understood as a pioneer in what is known as the history of ideas. This perspective is most welcome, as it is an overarching assumption of most of my sources that the idea of Cartesian Dualism has a special history, one that is very old and long-lasting, extending into current times. However, this book was published in 1928, and seems anachronistic to this understanding, for it reads like a triumphant obituary of this most hated idea. Needless to say, the pronouncement of death was premature.

Lovejoy (1955) writes to celebrate "the most characteristic and most ambitious philosophical effort of our generation." This effort was toward the victory against Descartes and Galileo, and optimism is high. "The occasion is being joyously celebrated in several quarters by the issuance of declarations of independence directed against those thinkers."

This political language is chosen quite deliberately. They are the "framers of. . . (Dualism's) constitutional law" and although there have been occasional "insurrections" up until that point, it is only then that there was enough "philosophical radicalism" to discard it altogether. Further, "from many sides" there are "rallying-cries" to "attack the common enemy," and many declare that "the enemy has in fact been already overthrown." Quoting a 1926 article, "the history of modern philosophy. . . is a history of the development of Cartesianism in its dual aspect of idealism and mechanism." Although there have been prior reservations, "only now have we begun to see in this simple and direct philosophy the source of all the great intellectual sophisms of our age." More than a few are "zealously engaged in attempts to emancipate philosophy" from this influence (pp. 1–3).

However, dualism is not so simple and direct, because the dualism is itself dual. For Lovejoy (1955), the interest is in the "attempt to escape from that double dualism" that those thinkers exemplified. The "double" in this case refers, on the one hand, to the epistemological dualism of representation, and on the other hand, to a "psychophysical dualism" concerning ontology. The latter is described as a "cleavage of the universe into two realms," or two worlds, which also have nothing in common; they are "mutually exclusive and utterly antithetic" (p. 3). "Against both dualisms, then, our age has witnessed an assault," the degree of which has never been seen "anywhere in the previous history of philosophy" (p. 4).

In spite of such strong rhetoric of victory, Lovejoy is dutiful enough to note a certain uneasiness in the proclamation of victory. That is, even in his own times, he also documents sources from other disciplines in which Cartesian influence is not rejected, but triumphantly celebrated. One example is from modern physics. Recall that Einstein and his theory of relativity was one of the transcenders, but for at least one of Lovejoy's (1955) early-century sources, relativity is seen as the natural continuation, and even completion, of Cartesian philosophy, and this is regarded as positive. Thus, Lovejoy notes a rather stunning irony. "Descartes has been dethroned; his sovereignty. . . decisively vindicated" (p. 6). The king is dead, long live the king.

Although Lovejoy (1955) spends most of his time in the book on the side of the happy victors, he correctly documents that this ambivalence is a significant unresolved problem in philosophy. A such, the following sentence has aged very well: "The past quarter century's discussion has shown that it is not easy for the critics of dualism to keep clearly in view its essential outlines" (p. 13). This line might well have been an epigraph to this book, although, I would have dropped the word "quarter." Further, he hints at what might be a central element in this unresolved problem. "Most of those who proclaim the obsolescence of 'Cartesian dualism' seem to have no sense of the fact that *such a task is incumbent on them*" [italics added]. Such difficult work appears to center on terminology regarding matter.

"The terms 'physical object' and 'physical event' must be given clear and consistent definitions" (p. 237). This is a crucially important suggestion that will be addressed later in this book.

The ghost in the machine

It is most likely from Ryle's (1966) *The Concept of Mind* that we get the image of the "ghost in the machine," which seems to come up frequently in contemporary discussions of Cartesian philosophy. According to Ryle (1966), this "doctrine. . . hails chiefly from Descartes" (p. 11), and that it "continues to distort" Western ideas of mind (p. 8). However, it is noted that this association has been more recently challenged by dedicated scholars (Cottingham, 1998, p. 21). Nonetheless, Ryle sees this influence as categorically destructive and injurious. As such, he states, "I shall often speak of it, with deliberate abusiveness" (p. 15), and that he wishes to "explode" it (p. 16). This is typical of the kind of emotions and overreaction that usually accompanies discussions of the Cartesian Split.

Also, Ryle frames almost every argument in terms of what can be called the *Two Worlds* view. It is important to understand this reference clearly because it may have been a foundational idea in Cartesian critiques. Many of my previous reference sources included some kind of a description of dualism in terms of two worlds. A deeper understanding of it will also serve as a useful point of orientation for much of the remaining investigation.

The Two Worlds view can be summarized as follows. This is the idea that, under Cartesian influence, modern people live in a "bifurcated" reality, living two different lives, and in two different worlds simultaneously (Ryle, 1966, p. 12). Baker and Morris (2002) outline four essential aspects of this view. First, there is an inner world of thoughts and other nonphysical mental objects. These all together form a kind of parallel world to the world of material objects. Second, mental objects include a wide range of various nonpropositional states of consciousness, such as "headache." Notably, this includes feelings and emotions. Excluded from this world are the processes of bodies and animals, which are nothing but unconscious clockwork. Third, inner objects are private and perceived by an infallible faculty of introspection. In an exactly opposite manner, outer objects are public, and perceived by the five external senses, although fallibly. Fourth, the inner and outer worlds interact via two-way causation (p. 7). The two worlds are therefore mirror opposites from each other, but still share a kinship of modality.

It can easily be seen how this view of reality is easily expressed by the image of the Ghost in the Machine. The Ghost is explicitly immaterial but operates in a way that is closely analogous to how material things work. In other words, the Ghost, or the mind, is understood to watch video monitors and pull on imaginary levers, in the brain, to operate the machinery of the body.

Respectfully, Ryle (1966) admits to, and defends, his emotional arguments against this Two Worlds view. The "heat" of his "excessively polemical" arguments style originates from his own feeling as a "victim" of it. He writes, therefore, from a place of liberation from this injurious influence, and wishes to share this result with others (p. 9). Ryle's conviction in this enterprise is noteworthy. What follows the introductory remarks can only be described as a sustained, almost militant logical attack, on multiple fronts.

Although his arguments are generally coherent and persuasive, what is lost in this approach is precision, at least in terms of etiology. A doctrine believed to be so universally destructive should have its origins carefully scrutinized. In this case, this should be a close attention to Descartes' writings, and ideally, locating these writings in historical and cultural context. Unfortunately, neither of these elements is present, apparently lost in the heat of the argument. Over 300 pages are dedicated to argument, without a single footnote or citation of any kind. Others have commented on this, quite disparagingly (Baker & Morris, 2002, p. 53). Unfortunately, this kind of treatment among critics is quite common.

Regardless, Ryle (1966) makes several interesting arguments that are worth consideration. In his view, Cartesian dualism is wrong not because of the separation of the two worlds, but because a conception of two worlds is incoherent to begin with. In other words, to even consider mind and matter as comparable "worlds" is what Ryle refers to as a category mistake. For Ryle, mind is a phenomenon that belongs to a completely different logical category than body. Thus, Cartesian Dualism, as Ryle understands it, tries to understand the two worlds as if they were of analogous structure, even if they are treated as polar opposites. This, for Ryle, is the big mistake, and is akin to confusing an abstract concept, such as team spirit, with an actual team member (pp. 16–17).

Ryle also makes a noteworthy point regarding Descartes' potential motivations, which might surprise some modern critics. As covered, it is common for people to loosely equate reductive mechanism with Cartesian dualism, or to view it as a necessary consequence of it. However, Ryle (1966) argues that Descartes, in spite of his scientific advances, was acting against such mechanism, when it came to the workings of the mind, or the soul. It was because he could not find an explanation for these things, using the budding mechanistic theories of his time, that he considered mind to be distinct from body. Overall, Ryle seems congenial to this motivation. However, he contends that Descartes' central mistake was to then draw analogies for this mental realm from those mechanistic models, even if they took the form of opposites (p. 19). This amounts to Descartes creating the Two Worlds view, inner versus outer. Although this overall interpretation has been questioned (Baker & Morris, 2002), I believe the point is worth considering, if only to highlight the tension between reductive mechanism and philosophical dualism, which are frequently conflated together by critics, as both being "Cartesian."

Overall, I consider Ryle's arguments to be mostly sound. The "dogma of the ghost in the machine" (Ryle, 1966, pp. 15–16) and its concomitant Two

Worlds view, is surely flawed, at least as a logical explanatory model for whatever the relationship is between mind and body. However, perhaps this "dogma" was never a logical model to begin with, as demonstrated by the tenuous link to its supposed creator, a point that will be explored more in later sections. For now, it is enough to suggest it is better understood as a myth than a model.

Ryle does in fact explicitly refer to it as a myth, but his usage of this term requires some exposition. In general, he uses it to primarily denote falsity. In other words, it *cannot be true* that the mind is to matter as a ghost is to a machine. However, the word *myth* can mean more than this. In the depth psychological tradition, a myth refers to something that is literally false, but psychologically true. A myth is a statement that refers to some aspect of reality, but that which is outside the boundary of conventional understanding. Because of this, it frequently appears in terms that are not literally true, but this itself is a true aspect of its necessary expression. In other words, a myth has to be literally false, in order to convey a sense of the unknown.

To his credit, Ryle (1966) does in fact leave some room for this notion, in his usage of the term. "A myth is, of course, not a fairy story," it may be referring to something real, but simply using the wrong terms (p. 8). Also, he recognizes that a myth may serve some kind of historical purpose, in terms of how a culture organizes its ideas over time. As such, the "two-worlds myth" may have been an improvement over older theological models, such as those in place during Descartes' time (pp. 23–24). However, Ryle is certain that this myth has outlived whatever usefulness it may have once had, and now is entirely false. By contrast, I argue the myth still has meaning, if understood properly. Specifically, it needs to be understood with archetypal depth. Of course, it is not literally true that we are ghosts in machines, but perhaps this is because it is mythically true, and remains so today. As such, logical debates against its various absurdities, such as the infinite regress, is likely to not have any lasting effect.

Finally, it seems that Ryle, for all his good points, is a fine example of many bad habits that frequently accompany debates against Cartesian dualism. Ryle pays no attention to Descartes' actual writings, he does not do full justice to context, and his polemics, although self-admitted, do not leave much room for critical reflection. It is noteworthy that contemporary arguments follow many of the same general patterns. And yet, even after over 60 years, many of these tendencies have expanded, and in some cases become even more dramatic, and less precise.

The masculinization of thought

Susan Bordo, however, is an exception to this overall trend. In her book *The Flight to Objectivity*, she plays close attention to the source material, and also views it in context. But her real project is for a new interpretation of the source texts, leading to a better understanding of contemporary concerns. For Bordo (1987), we are now experiencing a crisis of modernity (p. 2), and in order to better understand this, we need a better understanding of how it was originally formed. For this, she turns to Descartes and the *Meditations,* as a pivotal figure and text at the birth of the modern era. Bordo draws inspiration from several psychoanalytic perspectives, although she does not employ a personalistic reduction. That is, she rightly avoids the suspicion that Cartesian philosophy is wholly a product of problems related to Descartes' upbringing.

Bordo's (1987) approach is indeed novel. She argues that, after hundreds of years, the "pivotal philosophical texts of modernity" have not yet been read properly. They are still treated as abstract and disembodied philosophical arguments, rather than being placed in historical and cultural context (p. 2). Further, Bordo reads the *Meditations* in an embodied way. This may seem out of place, but Bordo rightly calls attention to the very strong images of profound anxiety, including psychosomatic disturbances, that are highly prevalent in the opening pages (p. 14). This kind of reading has been missing from conventional treatments.

Seen from this perspective, the *Meditations* is not a sourcebook for the supremely confident, rationalistic ego, but a symptom of cultural anxiety, in which something was tragically lost from the Middle Ages. This is then reflected in the unique, bodily reactions found in the *Meditations.* By understanding this, we can better respond to resultant anxieties today, in the postmodern age. For Bordo (1987), what was lost from the Middle Ages is a worldview in which an "organic female universe" was still present (p. 5), and also Hermetic science, which was more holistic and relational, than the modern era which subsequently "dethroned" it, with the overall "masculinization of thought" (p. 9). Such Cartesian anxiety, displayed in both the *Meditations* and in today's culture, represents a need to reintegrate those lost maternal values. Another noteworthy insight is that Bordo judges the *Meditations* to be more of a psychological work than philosophical one (p. 6).

I agree with Bordo that the *Meditations* has not been properly read. It has not been fully put in context, and its psychosomatic aspects have not been properly emphasized. However, I am suspicious of some of the historical presuppositions with which Bordo frames her new interpretation. For one, I am not entirely convinced that the Middle Ages were quite as healthy as she describes, in terms of the "organic female universe," and in having hermetic science as "enthroned." Although many in the patristic tradition employed such terms as the *anima mundi,* and also practiced astrology, many such practices were also condemned or disparaged. Alchemists were usually considered heretics. Further, in the *Summa Theologiae, Ia, q. 92, a. 1, Obj. 1.,* Aquinas entertains an argument from a contemporary that woman should never have been created in the first place, due to their imperfection (aquinasonline, n.d., paras. 2–4).

Another problem is that Bordo (1987), like Ryle, does not display much awareness of the mythological Descartes. That is, in spite of her disavowal of philosophy's tendency to repeat "clichés and sedimented emphases" (p. 2), she still falls prey to many of these same prejudices, especially in terms of understanding Descartes' writings in terms of the Two Worlds. Bordo frequently employs the terminology of a Cartesian "inner" world as something fundamentally distinct from the "outer" (pp. 7, 10), which is a schema that is really inherited from Ryle. She even frames the tragic dethronement in terms of the Two Worlds view. It is a "'drama of parturition': cultural birth out of the mother-world of the Middle Ages and Renaissance, and creation of another world — the modern" (p. 5).

Lastly, it is noted that the two worlds are now generally much further apart than in Ryle's. Bordo (1987) states that an "enormous gulf" now separates the "in here" from the "out there," and this leads to a position of deep alienation, because only God can "bridge the gulf between the 'inner' and the outer'" (p. 55). For Ryle, the two worlds are in mundane, constant interaction, as shown by the Ghost in the Machine. This is a kind of exaggeration that is commonly found outside of dedicated scholarship.

Cartesian disenchantment

The theme of Reduction and Isolation, when explored more deeply in other works, tends to drift toward a more commonly known theme, that of the so-called disenchantment of the modern era. This disenchantment is very often associated with the Scientific Revolution, and so it is natural that Descartes is mentioned as a founding figure. Even though there are many other potential figureheads, such as Newton, Bacon, and Galileo, Descartes is very often presented as a central figure of this development.

An exemplary work of this kind is a book by Morris Berman (1981), appropriately titled *The Reenchantment of the World*. Berman does indeed explore the specific contributions of those other historical figures, but Descartes is chosen as primary representative of modern disenchantment (p. 24). Berman defines this term as that of "nonparticipation," or that which insists on a "rigid distinction between observer and observed." Consciousness therefore becomes "alienated." "There is no ecstatic merger with nature, but rather total separation from it. Subject and object are always seen in opposition to each other" (pp. 16–17). Given this familiar rhetoric, it is no surprise that Berman's "disenchantment" becomes virtually synonymous with the adjective "Cartesian."

What is striking in Berman's treatment is the severity of the condition and the somewhat radical implications. Earlier I noted that he relates Cartesian dualism closely to mental illness, but the book explores other very negative connotations. Disenchantment is related to the self splitting into two; the mind retreats from the body, but observes it, in a cold, detached fashion. The mind regards the body as "false, or dead." Worse, "perception is thus unreal, and action correspondingly futile" (p. 19). This leads to more splitting, and a condition of numbness, suffocation, or "existential guilt" (p. 20). This condition has "destroyed the continuity of the human experience and the integrity of the human psyche. It has very nearly wrecked the planet as well" (p. 23). It results in a "spiritual vacuum," the loss of meaningful relationship with nature, the body, and the unconscious. Unless these can be recovered, "what it means to be a human being will forever be lost" (p. 132). Cartesian dualism leads to "the most unecological and self-destructive culture and personality type that the world has ever seen" (p. 189). The split within modern science "cannot be extended any further without the virtual end of the human race" (p. 193).

As with many other sources in this study, the intensity of such dramatic claims tends to overshadow the original subject, which is believed to be behind all the problems. In some respects, this seems to even preclude a proper understanding of it. Although Berman does spend some time with Descartes' texts, what he means specifically by "Cartesian" becomes almost meaningless under scrutiny. Berman (1981) himself seems to acknowledge this. He notes that "although the denial of participation lies at the heart of modern science, the Cartesian paradigm as followed in actual practice is riddled with participating consciousness" (p. 136). This seeming contradiction works throughout history as well. Newton's theory of gravity is at one time presented as being wholly anti-Cartesian, a complete rejection of Descartes' theory of vortices. And yet, since gravity is just another machine, "the central Cartesian outlook. . . was thoroughly validated by Newton's work" (p. 42). Later, the Cartesian program is identified with the goal of eliminating subjectivity. Even if this claim is granted, Berman notes the supreme irony that quantum mechanics establishes the opposite. Thus, the entire Cartesian enterprise to eliminate the subject ends up negating itself (p. 145). With all these contradictions, it is difficult to keep in mind a single definition of that which is causing the global calamity, so viscerally captured in other sections.

Beyond these difficulties, it is not even clear if the concept of disenchantment itself holds up under scrutiny. Josephson-Storm's (2017) *The Myth of Disenchantment* argues that the meaning of the term breaks down, both contemporarily and historically. In other words, with the growth of interest in various esoteric fields today, along with the widespread popular acceptance of astrology, we are arguably living in the most enchanting time period ever. Further, it turns out that the scientific luminaries who are often blamed for disenchantment were themselves steeped in occult practices. In other words, disenchantment is a modern myth, and yet a myth that captivates, and is often presented with new, mythic material. By this definition, it ironically negates itself as well, much like the entire Cartesian program. And this extends to other parts of Berman's book as well, with one section devoted entirely to the wisdom of alchemy. Thus, we are once again in uncertain territory, complex territory, as is fitting for a cultural complex.

The Cartesian mirror

The next work, Richard Rorty's (1980) seminal *Philosophy and the Mirror of Nature*, could arguably not count as a dedicated work, as it critiques the collective influence of three thinkers. Rorty argues that the legacy of Locke, Descartes, and Kant have bequeathed to us a particular notion of the pure intellectual mind, having of itself a "glassy essence," whose job it is to reflect on nature clearly, as a mirror would, and describe it fully. It is believed to be able to gradually work toward the ideal of understanding it perfectly. Regrettably, this idea of mind is now believed to be essential and universal, and we project it back onto the entire history of philosophy. Rorty argues, on the contrary, it is a local idea produced by those thinkers, and therefore it is highly contingent, rather than universal.

Regardless of the merits of this work, it becomes clear that Rorty (1980) spends more time with Descartes than the other two. Thus, what starts off as the "Descartes-Locke-Kant tradition," (pp. 8–9), gradually becomes the "Cartesian-Kantian pattern" (p. 9) or the "Cartesian-Kantian matrix" (p. 11), or the notion of an idea as "Cartesian-Lockean" (p. 28), but eventually becomes mostly about all things "Cartesian." Accordingly, the first page of the first chapter is specifically focused on Cartesian Dualism and its persistent, unique problems, still facing us today (p. 17). In this sense, it resembles closely the pattern I noted in the theme of the Dominant Paradigm, what can be called the pattern of the sub-Fathers. This was the pattern in which Descartes is both *the* Father and just another father at the same time.

The Cartesian theater

Daniel Dennett, referenced earlier as an ardent supporter of Damasio, wrote an influential book himself that certainly belongs in this inventory, titled *Consciousness Explained*. Dennett (1991) essentially takes up his argument where Ryle left off. Believing that Ryle successfully discredited the Ghost in the Machine, such that no self-respecting theorist today would ever openly espouse it, he argues that one remnant of it still remains in our theories, unconsciously and perniciously. That is, although the Ghost is banished, some residue of it remains in the common idea that there must be one special, central place in the brain, dubbed the "Cartesian Theater," where the mystery of self-awareness all comes together. For Dennett, this view seems satisfactory, but only because we assume it uncritically. Thus, his overall goal of the book is that of "toppling the dictatorial idea of the Cartesian Theater" (p. 171).

It is very interesting to note how Dennett (1991) regards the Cartesian Theater in terms of its seductiveness, such that it must be resisted by strong, disciplined minds. "All along the way we have to resist the alluring simplicities of the (Cartesian Theater), until we can secure ourselves on the new foundation" (p. 17). "It is one of the main burdens of this book to explain consciousness without ever giving in to the siren song of dualism" (p. 33). Unless we challenge ourselves, "the Cartesian Theater will continue to attract crowds of theorists transfixed by an illusion" (p. 39). "We must resist temptation; 'adopting' dualism is really just accepting defeat without admitting it" (p. 41). Many fall victim to this idea. Dennett details a current theory only for you to see whether you fell into the trap. He states, "if you find this conclusion compelling, you are still locked in the Cartesian Theater. A thought experiment will help you escape" (p. 115). The danger is always present. "It looks suspiciously as if we are drifting inexorably back to an internal Cartesian Self," yet there are still "some ways of escaping that dreadful denouement" (p. 219–220). For another common idea, he warns, "don't fall in the trap. This is our old nemesis, the Audience in the Cartesian Theater" (p. 445).

Thus, Dennett's (1991) account gives colorful illustration to the theme of the Tragic Transcender.

> Many theorists would insist that they have explicitly rejected such an obviously bad idea. But as we shall see, the persuasive imagery of the Cartesian Theater keeps coming back to haunt us — laypeople and scientists alike — even after its ghostly dualism has been denounced and exorcized.
>
> (p. 107)

One example is Wasserman, who seems to reject it, but "then goes on to fall in the Cartesian trap" (p. 164). To help present his own model, he exposes several other "experts tying themselves in knots because they are genuine Cartesian materialists in spite of themselves" (p. 139). He describes Cartesian Materialism as "the view that nobody espouses but almost everybody tends to think in terms of" (p. 144).

Of course, it helps to sell this narrative if the Cartesian Theater is imagined to be massively powerful. "Slowly but surely we've been chipping away at the idea of the Cartesian Theater. . . . Mere glancing blows, I fear; the Cartesian Theater is still standing, still exerting a tenacious pull on our imaginations" (Dennett, 1991, p. 303). Or, "this just shows the powerful gravitational force that the Cartesian Theater exerts on our imaginations" (p. 397). The lay person has little chance. "The limited resources of everyday language pull them inexorably toward the simplistic Boss of the Body, Ghost in the Machine, Audience in the Cartesian Theater model" (p. 424). Finally, for the best kind of tragedy, the idea has to have malicious overtones. It is "is the most tenacious bad idea bedeviling our attempts to think about consciousness" (p. 108).

All of this does little to limit Dennett's (1991) own pride in successfully transcending this all-powerful, malignant influence. "The astonishingly persistent conviction that there is a Cartesian Theater is the result of a variety of cognitive illusions that have now been exposed and explained" (p. 431). Although in other moments, he realizes that such a proclamation risks undercutting his own story. And so, he admits only partial victory. His version of neo-materialism promises a faithful account of consciousness, but only later, on "some sweet day," when we are finally able to "abandon more of Descartes's legacy" (p. 42). Further, "the Cartesian Theater will continue to haunt us until we have anchored our alternative firmly to the bedrock of empirical science" (p. 227).

Dennett's overall goal can be summarized as de-mystifying consciousness, which is fitting, considering the title of the book. He believes we have an irrational desire to maintain a notion that consciousness is special, unique, and cannot be explained away. He is not sympathetic to this view at all, seeing only intellectual laziness. His position could be paraphrased as: "There's no magic here, folks. Just lots and lots of neurons, doing their thing." But herein lies a most astounding irony. If there is no magic in this topic, one cannot help but wonder: How is it then possible that a quaint old idea from the 17th century could continue to haunt us? Worse, to be able to trap us, bedevil us, against our better will and judgment, requiring exorcism from experts? Nothing but a magical idea itself could have such a persistent effect. Dennett, in spite of his professed materialism, uses here the language of a spiritualist. With his constant warnings of the seductiveness of the diabolical Devil/Dualism, he almost comes across as a tent-pole evangelist. One can imagine such a figure, promising the miracle cure for our collective demonic possession, by slapping us on our foreheads, and shouting in front of the screaming masses: "Descartes, I call you out. Begone from this body!"

The turning point

If Dennett is an advocate for materialism, then Fritjof Capra's (1983) *The Turning Point* takes up an oppositional stance. However, as is often the case with this subject, they have their common enemy. In this case, in particular, this makes for very strange bedfellows indeed.

For Capra, similar to Berman, the label "Cartesian" generally resolves to anything associated with an outdated mechanistic worldview, and this is the primary subject matter of the book. What is most harmful of this view of reality, is that everything is seen as being composed of isolated, smaller bits of material stuff, which interact and behave according to exact mathematical laws. Complex phenomena must be broken down into these smaller parts in order for truth to be determined, and this is done analytically and rationally, with the goal of absolute certainty. In other words, this is the view of Dennett's materialism. Capra (1983) believes that although modern physics has largely abandoned this worldview, he argues that it remains pervasive and highly influential in practically everything else. As a result of this misunderstanding of reality, a "crisis of perception," we currently suffer from a wide variety of social and environmental ills (p. 15).

Capra's book is unique, however, because it takes up within it a wide variety of positions. Although generally reacting against mechanistic reduction, his stance occupies many different themes presented thus far, in a single work. It is doubtful that Capra is aware of the numerous problems this raises, having within it all the contradictory interpretations of Cartesian dualism. For all of the difficulty with Ryle's and Dennett's views, at least they have the benefit of being internally consistent. As I will show, Capra's conception of the Cartesian legacy does not feature this. However, this is a good thing, as it is a powerful single testament to the full range of the Cartesian Split complex, and so I will dedicate extra space for its various notions and their expressions.

In certain aspects, Capra frames his arguments in a way similar to Ryle's Two Worlds view. Capra (1983) states that Descartes established the inner world by rejecting the outer world and the body. The senses are judged to not give an accurate depiction of reality. Correspondingly, he only trusts the inner world, "the pure and attentive mind," characterized by intuition and deduction. "The essence of human nature is thought." He also emphasizes that "Cartesian" signifies a radical prioritization of inner over outer. Correspondingly, mind is more certain than matter, and mental work privileged over manual (p. 59). Further, not only is our identity essentially spiritual, but this inner world is where all the values are. Capra states that, for Descartes, "there was no purpose, life, or spirituality in matter" (p. 60).

However, Capra diverges from Ryle in terms of defining the nature of this inner world. Instead of consisting of all states of consciousness, including feelings and emotions, Capra (1983) defines the Cartesian inner world as intellectual thinking only, characterized by an exclusive emphasis on mathematics, logic, and clear and distinct reasoning (pp. 58–59). Defining the *cogito* along these lines is probably more prevalent among non-philosophical critiques of Descartes. However, this interpretation requires a neglect of certain prominent passages from Descartes, such as those that emphasize the role of sensation and emotion in the *cogito*.

A further and more significant problem arises when this inner world, consisting of rational thinking only, is then described in terms of how it relates to the outer world. In Ryle's view, the two worlds interact. However, in Capra's formulation, as in Bordo's, they are much further apart, suggesting that such a relationship is precluded at the very outset. Capra (1983) states that Descartes created a "fundamental division between two independent and separate realms" (p. 60). Again, they are "separate and fundamentally different" (p. 59). Finally, "mind and body belonged to two parallel but fundamentally different realms, each of which could be studied without reference to the other" (p. 166).

With this rhetoric of radical, fundamental separation, a new notion emerges. For Capra, the Cartesian inner world is rational thinking only, and there is no shortage of emphasis on how radically and completely it is split off from the outer world. When these two notions are synthesized, it essentially amounts to a position of solipsism. As summarized above, Capra's (1983) Descartes is solitary, sure of only his own existence, contemplating only his own thinking process, and is only certain of the thoughts that are carefully deduced from other thoughts, through a process of analysis (p. 58). *Radical isolation is then implied from the formerly established radical split between the two worlds.* There is no hope of ever being able to determine knowledge of the outer world, even through the senses, because it is presupposed from the start that it is fundamentally separate and independent. Cartesian rationality, combined with a radical Split, necessarily leads to what I call Cartesian Solipsism. This is not necessarily the same as philosophical solipsism, which concerns skepticism of other minds, although much has also been written on that subject in relation to Descartes. For the purpose of my research, however, it is noted only that Cartesian Solipsism denotes a condition of isolation from a separate material world, as well as loss of any knowledge of it. Sensation is no longer just doubtful, but now fundamentally impossible.

However, in other sections of the book, a new difficulty arises, for another version of Descartes can be discerned. Capra's (1983) other Descartes, in spite of his supposed radical dualism between two completely different realms, sees no problem with extending the range of certainty to the realm of matter as well, without any difficulty or methodological modifications. "Cartesian certainty is mathematical in its essential nature." And mathematics, which Descartes originally finds only in his mind, is now applied to all physical objects, even the entire universe (p. 58). This sudden re-alignment between the two worlds is seen most strikingly in terms of the role of sensation, which has now suddenly become trustworthy. In the original Two Worlds view, sense data is flawed and untrustworthy, and Capra's (1983) Solipsist Descartes, in certain sections, echoes this (p. 59). But in other sections, the certainty that was once reserved for the inner world is unproblematically extended to the outer world. Cartesian influence, which must be questioned, has "led us to assume that our senses create some kind of internal picture that is a faithful reproduction of reality" (p. 301).

This sudden and newfound faith in the senses, and in the senses only, is also demonstrated by Capra's (1983) brief sketch of Western history, in which the past 300 years amounted to a "new sensate period," which replaced the more idealistic period of the Middle Ages. In this new view, "matter alone is the ultimate reality." Elsewhere, Descartes is mentioned as one of the chief luminaries of this new materialistic worldview (pp. 31–32, p. 47). Again, this is a stark contradiction from the Solipsistic Descartes, in which analytical thinking is the only reality (p. 58). This new conception of Descartes the Materialist is also closely correlated with contemporary scientism. "The Cartesian belief in scientific truth is still widespread today" (p. 57).

As a correlate to this newly *over*valued outer world, the notions of reality formerly associated with inner world, once considered primary and absolute, are now significantly reduced. Instead of Ryle's Ghost in the Machine, which is actively pushing and pulling levers to make the body-machine move, Capra's (1983) materialistic Descartes now imagines the mind to be much smaller. We are all "isolated egos," which are too easily distracted by physicality, as indicated in the trends of consumerism and the search for the ideal body image (pp. 59–60). Our activities are limited to passively watching a stream of images, projected onto an inner mental screen, gathered from the outside by the senses (p. 295, p. 301). But because this is believed to be a sensate paradigm, these images are a faithful reflection of the ultimate reality. Certainty is established only from the scientific method (p. 58), which is primarily based on sensory data.

Thus, with extreme but apparently unnoticed irony, Descartes the Materialist is now thoroughly embedded in sensory images of the outer world, and has apparently lost any notion of a distinct inner world, the favored realm of the Solipsist. Also lost is any sense of the two worlds together, the position of Descartes the Dualist. In addition to the difficulty of managing now three different versions of Descartes, all of them are unfaithful reproductions of Descartes' actual writings. Also, somehow, all three versions, combining almost the entirety of a philosophical spectrum, are believed to be operating together in a single paradigm, which is understood to be shared by all, outside of a select few.

Capra also demonstrates the theme of the sub-Fathers. He delves into separate treatments of Galileo, Newton, and Bacon, and although they each had specific contributions toward the budding scientific age, Capra eventually considers all of them to be aspects of a single Cartesian idea. In the process, some important points are neglected.

Capra (1983) argues that it is actually Galileo who banished "merely subjective mental projections" from science, and this anticipated Descartes. It was Galileo who rejected from the sciences the senses, aesthetics, ethics, values, quality, form, feelings, motives, intentions, soul, consciousness, and spirit (p. 55). Regardless of the accuracy of this assessment, it is extremely ironic to note that the *Meditations* deal with these topics extensively.

Regarding Newton, Capra (1983) correctly notes that Newton's physics went far beyond Descartes' theories, and was the first to formulate a comprehensive and universal mathematical description of motion (p. 63). But Capra later goes on to describe Newton and his influence in an almost point-for-point parallel to what he had formerly described as the Cartesian paradigm (pp. 64–67). In other words, the dominant Newtonian paradigm is still Cartesian, in spite of Newton developing a much different, and more successful, physics.

Similarly, Capra also has his own inventory of Tragic Transcenders, in addition to those mentioned above in that section. In psychology, Spinoza and Leibniz both took up arms in refuting the Cartesian paradigm, substituting instead a "mystical monism" and windowless monads, respectively. However, each of these clearly failed to take hold (Capra, 1983, p. 167). In biology, there were a long line of new developments and new theories that all challenged Cartesian ideas, although somehow, Cartesian influence remained unscathed. This includes evolutionary theory (p. 72), the pioneering work of Galvani and Volta (p. 107), and the nondualism of La Mettrie (p. 107). Further, biological cell theory was a revolutionary step forward in biology and medicine in the 19th century. This was clearly quite removed from Descartes' antiquated physics, which featured the rapidly moving fine matter of "animal spirits." And yet, for Capra, simply because it seeks to explain all life processes in terms of fundamental units, this new belief "gave the Cartesian paradigm a new meaning" (p. 109). And, as referenced earlier, even Einstein tried to go beyond Descartes, but in the end, only reinforced the overall Cartesian program.

Capra's presentation of these Tragic Transcenders brings to life yet another version of Descartes. This version in particular grants an almost supernatural status to Descartes' legacy. But this is ironic, as Descartes was only a human being. A human being simply does not have the power to enforce a flawed ideology onto the entire history of modern thought.

On the other hand, Descartes the Evil Magician can. This Descartes was able to plant a seed of a bad idea in the entire Western psyche, with only ink and paper, and ensured that all subsequent geniuses would work fervently to bring his ultimate plan to fruition, even in spite of what seemed to be intentions to overcome it. The Cartesian idea, whatever it is, seems powerful enough to assimilate unto itself all subsequent developments in science, even as they all seem to present direct challenges to the entrenched Cartesian worldview.

Capra's overall aim is to challenge established systems of thought, and in this one respect, I consider it successful. However, his treatment of the influences on these systems, especially when using the label "Cartesian," is of course highly problematic. Also, it is noted that, similar to Ryle, Capra presents his arguments without a single direct quote from Descartes' actual writing. Again, this indicates a certain false sense of confidence, which is indicative of a complex.

At this point, I should emphatically state that I do not intend at all to disparage Capra's work. On the contrary, I find this book to be of extraordinary value, precisely because of the sometimes glaring inaccuracies and fantastic claims. As stated before, I consider the problem of Cartesian misinterpretation to be intrinsically meaningful, rather than a mere intellectual failure. Myths are singularly characterized by fantastic claims and seeming contradictions, and Capra's version is no different. Seen in this way, I consider this book to be a rich presentation of material that is highly relevant to a depth psychological study, if recognized as such.

The murder of the world soul

My final source in depth comes from my own field of depth psychology. Interestingly, there is really one source worth including, in spite of Descartes' supposed influence on the entirety of the Western mind. Freud appears to be mostly uninterested, having offered only one very scant interpretation of one of Descartes's famous dreams (Cole, 1992, pp. 11–13). Marie-Louise von Franz, a prominent first-generation Jungian, dedicates much more effort on the same subject but makes several critical errors (p. 233). In a previous work, I explore my own inventory of such errors and argue that she ends up dedicating most of the space to advance her own preferred theories, more than treating the original subject (Short, 2018, pp. 69–72). Also, Jung himself mentions Descartes very sparingly, and these evaluations are generally positive (pp. 64–68).

James Hillman, however, deserves special mention in this study. Although without a single dedicated work on the subject, others believe he perhaps should have made one. Olson (2013) states, "during the course of his life's work, Hillman has kept his focus on the achievement of a single, critical objective: to provide an archetypal corrective to a modern Cartesian consciousness that pervades every aspect of American culture" (p. 62). Similarly, biographer Dick Russell (2013) states, "Hillman would come to consider Descartes an arch-enemy, for having 'banished the psyche at the beginning of the modern period'" (p. 210).

For Hillman's own words, it is useful to start with his most influential book, *Re-Visioning Psychology,* which, fittingly, begins with Descartes. The first page of this seminal work lays out a grand, almost mythic context for his intended mission. Hillman (1992b) critiques modern psychology, whose basic modern view is the psychology of Descartes: "A universe divided into living subjects and dead objects. There is no space for anything intermediate, ambiguous, and metaphorical." Hillman intends to add the missing third perspective, that of soul, which essentially amounts to entering into another "psychological dimension" (p. 1).

Hillman is noteworthy in the history of psychology for many reasons, but one of which is his attention to detail on philosophy. Generally, he displays a wide familiarity with the history of philosophical ideas, and how these contribute to developments in contemporary psychology. Although his overall competence in this area seems to be sufficient, things tend to break down rather dramatically with his understanding of Descartes. In short, he tends to portray Descartes the Materialist, or more of an empiricist than a rationalist, and this is strikingly out of step of the most prominent commentary (Short, 2018, pp. 73–77). Thus, I consider it particularly meaningful when the philosophical Hillman makes this basic mistake regarding *the* central philosophical figure, both of his psychology, and of our entire culture. To my mind, it seems to highlight a central notion of my hypothesis, that is, whatever the Cartesian Split complex is, *it is best understood as a myth and not as a philosophy.*

Once this shift is allowed, Hillman's unique voice is a boon toward our understanding of the Cartesian Split complex. His rhetoric, even if sometimes loose and prone to mistakes, is, by any standard, vividly colorful and imaginative, and therefore meaningful. Hillman's presentation of the problem is, in his own words, a mythic vision, "a universe divided," and Descartes is the arch-enemy who rules over it.

Hillman offers plenty of other examples along these lines. "Cartesians. . . . abetted the murder of the world's soul" (Hillman, 1992a, p. 107). Descartes is also one of the four horsemen of the apocalypse, an apocalypse that "kills the soul of the world," and worse, is still happening now (p. 125). However, Descartes appears not only at the end of the world, but at the beginning as well, where he looms larger than life, assuming godlike, Biblical proportions. "The Earth had already been quite flattened by Western philosophy's first supreme developer, René Descartes (1596–1650) who named the world of material things—rocks and trees and our daily bread—*res extensa*" (Hillman, 2007, p. 321). But this is an evil god as well, requiring humans to seek salvation. Modern distractions "keep us in the Cartesian cemetery, flat and soulless, and gives over the world to the Christian Devil so we must pray to be risen from it" (p. 334). Also, this Descartes is also a Magician, who was somehow able to conjure up a spell to "banish the psyche" to the pineal gland, once again, "at the beginning of our modern period" (Hillman, 1992b, p. 10). He was even powerful enough to lay devious psychological snares, keeping minds trapped within error, even as they attempt to transcend it (pp. 116, 171). Of course, none of these references are best taken literally. Rather, they are a uniquely rich set of metaphors. However, I am not yet aware of any attempt to take these images seriously *and* metaphorically.

It remains to be seen if Hillman was ultimately successfully in his "single, critical objective" to overcome Descartes. Given the long list of Heroic Transcenders, who all failed in the end, I have my doubts. However, Hillman leaves two important contributions. The first is his emphasis on psychological image, which I am following in this study. I believe I am fortuitously applying this approach to Hillman's own understanding of Descartes, even if it is flawed. Or rather, perhaps because it is flawed, the image stands out more clearly, especially with the benefit of his rich and metaphorical prose.

In any case, Hillman's critique certainly leaves a legacy of Descartes that is more mythical than philosophical.

Second, it is a real gift to notice that the opportunity to delve deeper into the Cartesian Split is both pleaded for, and missed, in the very first pages of *Re-Visioning Psychology.* Hillman (1992b) writes,

> it's not, after all, Descartes's life we go on fighting, for Descartes is dead, although not his *Method,* nor his *Meditations.* That's where he lives. To find the author go to the book. If the author is anywhere, he's in the book, *is* the book.
>
> (p. x)

Unfortunately, like many others, Hillman does not go to the book, in this seminal work of archetypal psychology. There are no direct quotes, no footnotes, neither the *Method* nor *Meditations* are in the bibliography, and there are very good reasons to assume that Hillman has not read a single word of them since his undergraduate years. But for all this, he creates another book, a significant one. These quotes culled from his various works constitute, in my mind, the first stylistically complete presentation of the myth of the Cartesian Split.

Further evaluation

Hillman's rhetoric is but the capstone of many voices. I have included thus far well over 100 sources, but I could have included thousands. It is hard to get a group of scholars to agree on anything; it is in their nature to critique and dissent. But in this case, there is an odd consensus: Cartesian Dualism is a very bad idea and has been so for centuries. And yet, this consensus is still obviously too vague.

The Cartesian Split is discussed by so many authors in so many different ways, it is difficult to focus on it properly. Some will argue against Descartes the Dualist, in the manner of Damasio and Dennett, and others will argue against Descartes the Reductionist, in the manner of Berman and Capra. However, both argue exclusively rationally, and therefore in a one-sided manner. As long as these aspects are divided, the mythic elements are not recognized, and therefore the symbolic approach is precluded at the outset. It has been the goal of the last two chapters to consolidate much of these conflicting reports into a single location. Hopefully, this confluence of odd bedfellows makes it easier to see how this story is rich with potential meaning.

More pointedly, I hope this last approach has brought to life four unique versions of Descartes that are not readily found in the traditional philosophical literature. The first of these is the Radical Dualist, in which the two worlds do not interact. But there is also the Solipsist, who cannot even conceive of the material world, and its opposite on the other side, the Materialist, who cannot grant the reality of the immaterial world. And lastly, there is now the Evil Genius, who somehow is orchestrating it all.

It should also be noted that all of these new versions are direct descendants of the original Two Worlds myth, even if they seem to depart in opposite directions. It seems this happens as follows: First, the two worlds are created and separated, as in Radical Dualism. Then, one of those worlds completely eclipses the other, depending on which one is being emphasized at the moment. In this way, we are all Solipsists and Materialists at the same time, but unable to bridge the gulf, because we cannot even see it. And only an Evil Genius, employing a magic spell, can ensure that this paradoxical condition remains the single dominant worldview, uncritically accepted by all.

Worse, this worldview shows no sign of abating and is believed to be leading us to all sorts of urgent crises, in all facets of our civilization. This includes the economy, energy, health care, the environment, and even violent crime (Capra, 1983, p. 15). "The survival of our whole civilization" may depend on overcoming Cartesian influence (pp. 17–18).

Whether he intends or not, Capra's words, as well as Hillman's, invokes a mythic perspective. And this perspective invites a few more difficult questions. If geniuses such as Einstein could not wrest themselves free from this all-powerful and malignant spell, what possible hope can we have that the general population can succeed where they failed? If magic is involved, it is further doubtful that our secular society can properly defend itself. And even if we could collectively charm our way out of this curse, can it be done in time to preserve civilization? There appears to be no hope. We are living in the Myth of the Inevitable Cartesian Apocalypse.

When reflecting on this, one cannot help but reflect on the magnitude of the problem, signified by the Cartesian Split, which becomes truly mythic in scope. Such a far-reaching influence, encompassing entire philosophical spectrums, assimilating all modern developments, and which is now threatening the survival of our entire civilization, cannot be the result of a single human being. It can only be the result of unconscious forces in the psyche, which artificially constructs extraordinary stories out of mundane reality. These forces have been known to most human societies since the beginning of time, and have always been attributed to non-human entities. In short, what is holding us back in this divided, clockwork universe, which we seem unconsciously compelled to destroy, along with ourselves, *can be nothing less than a god*.

In this sense, all the dutiful recorders of the life and deeds of the Tragic Transcenders are absolutely right. Our best thinkers cannot extricate themselves from the Cartesian worldview, because they have been mistakenly arguing against Descartes, with or without the source texts. So long as the problem comes from a frail French philosopher who died almost 400 years ago, we will never understand its true nature, which, on the contrary, lives on in the depths of the psyche today.

References

aquinasonline. (n.d.). Retrieved June 1, 2016, from: http://www.aquinasonline.com/Questions/women.html

Baker, G. P., & Morris, K. J. (2002). *Descartes' dualism*. New York, NY: Routledge.

Berman, M. (1981). *The reenchantment of the world*. Ithaca, NY: Cornell University Press.

Bordo, S. (1987). *The flight to objectivity: Essays on Cartesianism and culture*. New York: State University of New York Press.

Capra, F. (1983). *The turning point: Science, society, and the rising culture*. Toronto, Canada and New York, NY: Bantam Books.

Cole, J. R. (1992). *The Olympian dreams and youthful rebellion of René Descartes*. Chicago, IL: University of Illinois Press.

Cottingham, J. (1998). Introduction. In J. Cottingham (Ed.), *Descartes* (pp. 1–27). New York, NY: Oxford University Press.

Dennett, D. (1991). *Consciousness explained*. Boston, MA: Back Bay Books.

Hillman, J. (1992a). Anima mundi: The return of the soul to the world. In J. Hillman (Ed.), *The thought of the heart and the soul of the world* (pp. 89–130). Dallas, TX: Spring.

Hillman, J. (1992b). *Re-visioning psychology*. New York, NY: Harper Perennial.

Hillman, J. (2007). Apollo, dream, reality. In J. Hillman (Ed.), *Mythic figures* (pp. 320–335). Putnam, CT: Spring.

Josephson-Storm, J. A. (2017). *The myth of disenchantment: Magic, modernity, and the birth of the human sciences* (1st ed.). Chicago, IL: University of Chicago Press.

Lovejoy, A. O. (1955). *The revolt against dualism: An inquiry concerning the existence of ideas*. LaSalle, IL: Open Court Publishing.

Olson, R. (2013). Psyche as postmodern condition: The situation of metaphor in James Hillman's archetypal psychology. *Janus Head*, *13*(12), 61–91.

Rorty, R. (1980). *Philosophy and the mirror of nature*. Princeton, NJ: Princeton University Press.

Russell, D. (2013). *The life and ideas of James Hillman*. New York, NY: Helios Press.

Ryle, G. (1966). *The concept of mind*. London, UK: Hutchinson's.

Short, B. (2018). *The depths of the Cartesian split: A hidden myth in modern psychology* (10822143) [Doctoral dissertation]. Pacifica Graduate Institute.

Chapter 4

Confronting the legend

The Cartesian Split certainly has a dubious history, but it is potentially even more dangerous if we cannot properly conceive of it. In the hypothetical case study, the fantastical stories of Rand's misdeeds have rendered Ash unable to properly function. There is in this a central problem, which must be addressed. There is no differentiation between the stories of Rand and Rand's actual life. The result of this is that Ash is perpetually a victim of monstrous deeds that occurred in the past, which may in fact have never happened. Until Ash comes to terms with the idea that Rand's stories are really Ash's stories, they will forever exert their influence, from the deep past, which can never change. A breakthrough occurs in therapy when Ash realizes that the stories were constructed, and perhaps are still being constructed, in the present moment. The story must be confronted as such.

This lack of differentiation has occurred, in varying degrees, in all of the authors mentioned thus far, with the general equation of "Cartesian" with Descartes. In contrast, there is a relatively small tradition in academic philosophy that has become aware of this problem; that our stories of Descartes are not the same as Descartes. It is what could be called "the Descartes Problem." Although I see the problem as a complex, the theorists I will now review do not use that terminology specifically, although they do in some cases describe it in roughly equivalent terms.

Paley (2002) has dedicated an entire essay to this overall problem. However, he is certainly not alone in having noticed the various ironies, misunderstandings, and impressive distortions of philosophical views that frequently accompany discussions of Cartesian dualism. In fact, this article seems to be a culmination of a slowly building awareness, within the field of academic philosophy, over the past four decades. I will now attempt to summarize this development.

First, it must be stated that I cannot possibly be comprehensive in my account. The sheer breadth of scholarly work on Descartes is much too large for an adequate survey, even for dedicated Cartesian scholars (Bracken, 2002, p. vii). As such, I can only hope to provide a rough sketch of this one single strand of thought in this tradition. Even so, I believe the strand I can identify is relatively contiguous and coherent. It is, again, the growing awareness of a pronounced divergence between the overall label "Cartesian" and the actual writings of Descartes. This development, as far as I am aware, has been centered in, and only in, the field of Cartesian scholarship.

The dawn of awareness

Three essays were published in the 1970s that seem to present a dawning consciousness of the divergence. The authors were mostly writing for their contemporaries. Surely, there are precedents to these examples, of which I am not familiar, but these will suffice for the points I need to make. The sentiment in these essays could be paraphrased as follows: "There seems to be some confusion with what Descartes actually wrote."

Margaret Wilson (1998) explores in detail the epistemological function of Descartes' distinction between mind and body. She frames her argument with an overall concern she has for a developing divergence in understanding. She states that, in spite of heavy philosophic discussion on Descartes' mind-body distinction, there has been "surprisingly little serious effort to gain an actual understanding of his position" (p. 186). She observes that Descartes' epistemological argument "has not been correctly represented or criticized" (p. 186). By contrast, there is a newly divergent opinion that Descartes' argument was primarily ontological, which is seen in all the discussions of Descartes' so-called substance dualism. In other words, a more substance-orientated Descartes has been born, one that separates reality, instead of seeking truth. Accordingly, Wilson is dutiful to use the word *distinction*, as opposed to the word *separation*, in reference to his dualism, as Descartes himself does.

John Cottingham (1998a) takes up the task of evaluating the claim that Descartes was unusually cruel to animals in his philosophy. There is a commonly held "monstrous thesis" that Descartes resolutely denied any and all feelings in animals. It is believed that Descartes provided "a grim foretaste of a mechanically minded age," which violated "the old kindly fellowship of living things" (p. 225). However, after a close analysis of Descartes' actual writings, "it is by no means clear" how this thesis is derived (p. 225). Cottingham suggests the problem lies with the frequent mistranslation of the word *cogitatio* into "experience," when for him, it is better translated as "awareness." In other words, Descartes could be understood as saying that an animal simply does not have reflective self-awareness of its feelings, while still experiencing the feelings themselves (p. 229). This seems to be not that controversial and is also not that far from the old scholastic conception of animals as lacking a rational soul (p. 228).

Jonathan Bennett (1998) discusses the tension between Descartes' dualistic conception of mind and body, which is claimed to be absolute, and other areas of his writing, in which he claims that all truths are dependent on God. Under standard Cartesian interpretations, these two positions are irreconcilable (p. 161). This text is interesting because Bennett is aware of a tendency of Cartesian scholars to marginalize certain difficulties or otherwise justify them. In his words, this tendency is "charitably shielding Descartes from his own splatter" (p. 160). I infer from this claim that two groups had slowly emerged within Cartesian scholarship, those that are enthusiastically critical of perceived problems, and those that are more or less apologists. Bennett seems wary of the latter; however, he takes up a subtle position and avoids being placed firmly in either. He states, "either [Descartes] had a blind spot in this direction, or we have misunderstood his doctrine about necessary truths" (p. 161). Bennett then proceeds with a different interpretation of necessary truths, one derived from the actual texts, and suddenly, a new Descartes emerges. This new Descartes is surprisingly self-consistent and in no need of an apologist. Bennett is "struck by how little my Descartes has to apologize for" (p. 162).

In summary, these three texts seem to highlight a developing tension between standard conceptions and the actual writings. In other words, there is another version of Descartes forming in the philosophic discourse, one that is slowly becoming out of step with his actual writings. This version of Descartes separates reality more than finding truth, is cruel to animals, and is internally inconsistent, but all of these positions are not clearly derived from the actual texts.

Bennett takes a crucial additional step, in noting that we may sometimes have to take on the responsibility for our own interpretations of the texts. There is a definite possibility here of Jungian shadow projection. If we have a vehement objection to Descartes, we must consider the possibility of projecting our own problems onto the text. More recently, others have also suggested this, more articulately (Baker & Morris, 2002, p. 2; Lee, 2013, p. 9). Consistent with projection, it may be more comforting to abide by standard interpretations, even if they are problematic, simply because it saves us the difficulty of questioning them in ourselves. This leads directly to the next stage of awareness.

The problem of interpretation

The next three essays were written in the 1990s, and seem to present a more articulate consciousness of severe problems with standard interpretations. Such interpretations now appear to be much too simple and limiting. In other words, Descartes the writer suddenly is revealed to be much more complex than standard interpretations have previously allowed. It is altogether remarkable, that after centuries of Cartesian scholarship, professionals are still struggling with such questions. What is new in these particular writings is that philosophers are now taking up a sense of responsibility, or acknowledgment of difficulty, in their present task of understanding

Descartes, perhaps following Bennett. This stage could be paraphrased as: "This confusion is creating a problem, and maybe the problem is us."

Daniel Garber (1998) examines the textual evidence for Descartes' role as a dutiful experimenter. This presents a problem because standard interpretations have placed Descartes firmly in the rationalist category, in which all truths come from the intellect. This is opposed to an experimentalist, in which knowledge comes from experience. To modern eyes, this "looks a bit puzzling" (p. 234). How can he be both at the same time? Garber then examines the text closely and concludes that the problem is in us. Descartes is simply both, but in order to see this, we must first abandon our preference for overly simplistic categories. "On the standard view of things. . . there are two sorts of philosophers: rationalists and empiricists." Once we see the evidence for Descartes the empiricist, "there is a temptation simply to think that Descartes must have been placed in the wrong slot." However, close textual analysis of Descartes the writer "reveals how crude the scheme of classification really is" (p. 258). In other words, attention to detail reveals how much more nuanced the overall situation really is, and that our own prejudices may be creating the problems.

Peter Markie (1998) discusses the *cogito* argument and its importance. Interestingly, he starts off with a standard interpretation of Descartes, clearly aware that it is far too simple, and in need of deeper understanding. He indicates this with the opening statement: "The basic story is well known." Descartes starts with doubting his senses and establishes certainty based solely on his own thinking, his existence. This doctrine seems "obvious" and "uninteresting," and in a sense, not even very original, as "St. Augustine anticipates him." However, things get more complex upon close reading. "Once we get beyond a superficial reading of the text," this claim of certainty becomes much more confusing (p. 51). Markie then wrestles with a new interpretation, one that seems more promising, but no final answers are given. Also, Descartes himself now actually appears as a present participant. In other words, Descartes is not discussed in terms of his age-old answers to questions, whether right or wrong, but more with raising important questions that still haunt us today (p. 77).

Roger Ariew (1992) challenges the standard view that Descartes established a firmly anti-scholastic position. To support this claim, scholars in the past have simply compared Cartesian and scholastic doctrines, side by side. Ariew claims that this is not sufficient. In order to properly understand Descartes' positions, we must take up the task of exploring his possible reasons for him taking such a position. Also, these reasons must be put in proper context (p. 58). Ariew finds new evidence in Descartes' correspondences that indicates he was not entirely antagonist to his formal education (pp. 61–62). The resultant image of Descartes is not the modern one, one that "dealt the final blow" to scholasticism (p. 80). Rather, the new image is more complex: One who carefully picked his battles, one thought at a time, rejecting some held truths while maintaining others, but always relying on reason, rather than dogma (p. 81). This would be a good model for anyone working in academia today, including staunch critics of Descartes.

In summary, these three works all start with a recognition that Descartes has suddenly become more nuanced, with more unnoticed subtleties, than standard interpretations previously allowed. Also, this awareness forms the impetus for a need to take on more responsibility for philosophical work today. There is also a notion that by reading Descartes, we can become aware of our own simplistic narratives that need to be challenged, as well as becoming more aware of the historical Descartes. However, in these works, there is still a general feeling that the standard interpretations, however partial, are at least faithful representations of at least something in Descartes' writings.

The problem of caricature

These next group of writings, by contrast, use language that indicates an awareness of a more extreme divergence. Now, standard interpretations are seen as gross mischaracterizations, or in some cases, as starkly incompatible with Descartes' actual writings. There is a new tone of subtle sarcasm toward naively held standard interpretations, which now appear to be seriously flawed, and completely ungrounded. The paraphrased sentiment could now be called: "OK people, this is starting to get silly."

Cottingham (1992), in an introductory essay, uses the word "caricature" to describe the increasingly large divergence between "Cartesian" and Descartes. He argues that close textual analysis reveals that Descartes' philosophy is actually "very far from matching the caricature of 'rationalist foundationalism' with which it is so often identified" (p. 2). It is commonly assumed that modern scientific approaches to consciousness are fundamentally Cartesian, but Cottingham states that Descartes' actual writings are "markedly out of step" with this (p. 10). Interestingly, the caricature may not be an entirely modern construction. He finds it also in Voltaire's historical criticism of Descartes (p. 18).

Cottingham (1998b) later wrote another introductory essay, in which the irony is highlighted more prevalently and forcefully. He starts with the taut observation: Descartes' reputation today is "strangely ambivalent," as he is both revered and reviled at the same time, but now, mostly reviled. The word "'Cartesian', by the end of the twentieth century, has for many philosophers become almost a term of abuse." As an example of this, Cottingham footnotes a very revealing 1995 quote from Kenny:

> Frege exposed Cartesian errors about thought while retaining. . . Cartesian errors about ideas. It is as if the residual poison running

> through the philosophical systems of the day was gathered by Frege. . . into a single virulent boil ready to be lanced by Wittgenstein.
>
> (p. 1)

This is another good example of both the Heroic and Tragic Transcender.

Cottingham (1998b) goes on to illuminate a highly irrational aspect of the perceived Cartesian legacy in Western philosophy. He does this by comparing to an analogous development, that of Galileo's legacy in the history of science. Galileo's physics is outdated, but nobody in science spends any time debating Galileo. Rather, he is briefly celebrated for what he got right, and the rest is uncontroversially discarded. However, with Descartes and philosophy, "things are very different." First, there are still a few (but only a few) philosophers today who might fairly be called "Cartesian." Second, Descartes' doctrines are not treated as merely historical curiosities. Rather, "some of the twentieth century's most original thinkers have expended vast amounts of energy in combating them" (p. 2). However, in spite of this effort, "contemporary philosophy feels compelled to insist on its emancipation from Cartesian paradigms" (p. 7). Third, regardless of the veracity of Descartes' claims, he established the very structure of the philosophical agenda for the next 350 years, enduring even today (p. 2). Clearly, Wittgenstein was unsuccessful in inoculating us from the residual Cartesian poison.

To the second point above, I would like to add a corollary. Although Descartes made significant contributions toward the developing scientific theories of the time, some of his ideas sound completely foreign to our modern sensibility. Descartes theorized that vacuums are impossible and that all events in space are caused by spinning vortices of very fine matter. However, these strange notions were quickly replaced by the more sophisticated theories of Newton and were soon completely discarded. Given this, one wonders why Descartes' philosophical ideas, which might be argued to be just as flawed and nonsensical, if not more so, are not only still being discussed, but believed to be the dominant paradigm. Perhaps he was simply a very persuasive writer, but if so, surely he would have employed those same skills toward his scientific ideas. So, there is a very strong asymmetry here, the reasons for which are not obvious.

Cottingham (1998b) also critiques the assumption that Descartes regarded the human being as comprised of two entirely distinct substances, mind and body. As we have seen, the image for this is the Ghost in the Machine. However, in Descartes' actual writings, according to Cottingham, we see the human being presented as a "real substantial union," a mysterious third thing that arises from the mutual intermingling of mind and body. The key phenomena that reveal this union are sensations, emotions, and passions, which are not reducible to either (p. 7). Also, this third thing cannot be intellectually understood, but rather, better to be experienced (pp. 19–20). According to Cottingham, philosophers "have often tended to ignore" these theories (p. 19).

By contrast, Genevieve Rodis-Lewis (1998) explores Descartes theories of mind-body union in detail. Aware of the significant divergence between these and the standard "Cartesian" model, she opens with slightly sardonic observation: "Descartes is often accused nowadays of having destroyed the unity of the human being" (p. 197). She then exposes in textual detail how Descartes the writer could never have held this view. Descartes "always affirmed the substantial union of soul and body" (p. 204). More interestingly, she shows that a Platonic inspired mind-body dualism was present well before Descartes, and his work was distinct to even these accepted doctrines (pp. 201–202).

Consonant with this, Amelie O. Rorty (1992) emphasizes how much importance Descartes the writer attributed to having a sound body. Employing the same terminology as Cottingham, Rorty recognizes that the common conception of Descartes in this regard is a caricature; however, this one is "grossly simplified" and "grotesque" (p. 371). In some cases, the caricature is merely an exaggeration, in other cases, a complete reversal. Contrary to the Platonic image of the privileged and infallible mind over the confused body (p. 371), Descartes, at times, actually proposes the opposite (p. 372). Although he was relentlessly optimistic about the power of the will, "Descartes nevertheless also shows how will depends on the cooperation of the body to correct or check its deviations" (p. 384). Rorty surmises that perhaps an excessive reliance on Descartes' writings on the will has led to the numerous "parody clichés about Descartes' pure intellectualism" (p. 384).

Rafaella De Rosa (2007) argues against the "standard" interpretation of Cartesian bodily sensations as nonrelational, qualitative experiences only, and of no help in determining the truth. This seems to fit the image of the "Rationalist Descartes." However, this argument is not his legacy. Further, there is strong textual evidence that he could not have held this view (p. 182).

The essays mentioned here have demonstrated a growing awareness that something has gone very wrong with standard interpretations, at times bordering on the absurd, or even the opposite of what Descartes actually wrote. However, this awareness is usually limited to introductions, as a framing device to allow the author to present a more faithful interpretation of Descartes. Other times, the divergence is simply noted for its absurdity, with the occasional witty side comment, parenthetical, or footnote. This growing awareness presents a new danger. In the previous chapters, I emphasized the reality of the Cartesian myth. However, with these treatments of absurdity, the mythical Descartes is in danger of being rationalized out of existence.

The reality of the problem

A survey of more yet recent literature, however, demonstrates yet another level of understanding of all this, and that is what seems to be a truly psychological, even a depth psychological layer. Rather than seeing the overall caricature of Descartes as a gross error, or source of amusement, certain philosophers have begun to see it as something quite serious, requiring its own explanation. It is no longer simply an expository or framing device, but as a subject worthy of investigation of its own right, at times, a psychological investigation. These selected works could be paraphrased as: "Western academia, you have a Cartesian complex. We need to talk about this."

One small example of this is Cottingham's (1998b) newer commentary on his own older essay on Descartes' treatment of animals. Here, he now makes a more striking, and more psychological, summation of his conclusion. Whereas before he was content to understand the "monstrous thesis" as perhaps a relatively innocent exaggeration, he now suggests it may be something more of an irrational defense mechanism. People today have become "more Cartesian than Descartes himself," and may be looking to absolve themselves of guilt, by hanging everything on Descartes (p. 22).

Harry Bracken (2002) opens his book on Descartes with a striking summary of the problem. Descartes has been "attacked, reviled, and condemned like no other thinker for most of the last 350 years. . . Refutations continue to pile up. European philosophy is haunted by Descartes and his ideas" (p. 1). He devotes an entire chapter trying to understand the reasons behind all the unwarranted, irrational, and unsubstantiated criticism. He asks, quite simply, "why is Descartes *the philosopher philosophers love to hate*?" (p. vii). Further, he acknowledges the emotional content that is frequently invoked whenever the subject of Cartesian dualism is approached, and what is usually neglected or ignored as a result (p. 21).

Robert Bolton (1999) argues that the rampant anti-Cartesianism over the past century can be seen as a kind of irrational reaction formation, and asks the simple question: To what extent is this reaction justified? He answers in the negative, and that the reaction may have unconscious psychological roots. This may be to protect us from our own bad habits of thinking, as well as to perhaps reassure us with an overly simplistic conception of reality, even if this not rationally defensible. Also, he recognizes that popular critiques assign far too much power to Descartes, in that the ability to force the masses to believe in a bad theory is usually reserved for supernormal or religious figures, not philosophers (para. 3–5). This is a point that I have of course been strongly emphasizing.

Tom Sorell (2005), in the introduction to his book, *Descartes Reinvented*, outlines a similar, but novel approach. First, Sorell starts out with the idea of the divergence as axiomatic. "The vilified Descartes of twentieth- and twenty-first-century philosophy is not the same as the canonical Descartes." However, Sorell goes further, and distinguishes a third Descartes, the historical Descartes, the Descartes of the "best informed specialists," the Descartes who slowly emerges through critical, contextual studies in the history of philosophy. This leaves the canonical Descartes as simply the words on the page. All three have "legitimate philosophical roles." What is particularly interesting is that Sorell accepts an inherent risk to the interpretive process. That is, trying to understand Descartes seems to necessarily carry the risk of producing a distortion, in this case the vilified Descartes. But this very process is how philosophy is desired to help solve contemporary issues. "Caricature is tolerable for the sake of relevance" (p. xx). In other words, by continuing to discuss Descartes with contemporary problems in mind, new philosophical problems are being worked out, even if we haphazardly construct a villainous Descartes. Sorell therefore appreciates the reality of the vilified Descartes, while at the same time critiquing it. He wants to honor it as part of a larger process, while at the same time, emphasizing the importance and relevance of the canonical and historical Descartes.

Another work which dwells significantly on the Descartes Problem is *Reading Descartes Otherwise*, by Kyoo Lee (2013). Lee, like Sorell, takes the divergence to be axiomatic: "Whatever or whoever we think he is, he says he is not *that*" (p. 3). Lee puts forth her own case for a re-reading of the original texts. In Lee's interpretation, following Bordo, we do not find the traditional Descartes at all. Contrary to the rationalistic and supremely confident version, we instead find a lone and solitary "thinker," beset on all sides by a terrifying landscape of doubt and impending madness. Also, we see "borderline cases of psychosomatic disorder," which call into deep question the very structure of identity. In short, under Lee's reading, the *Meditations* becomes a psychological drama, one that can still be intriguing and relevant for us today.

In Paley's (2002) essay, he highlights some of the deeply irrational beliefs that are exposed once one closely examines the arguments against anything "Cartesian." Although his focus is on nursing philosophy, I believe his observations have much wider applicability. Following Bracken's lead, he notes a fundamental paradox at the heart of "Descartes-bashing." He asks,

> if the hostility to Descartes has been so widespread for so long, in what sense has he been influential? How can it be said that Cartesianism permeates the modern world if virtually no-one has had a good word to say about it?
>
> (p. 1)

Paley's argument is loose, rhetorical, and at times exaggerated, but seems highly appropriate for the subject. He ponders the question: Is Descartes capable of controlling our thoughts from beyond the grave, making us believe in his terribly flawed ideas, infecting our schools, despite all the best efforts of our intellectual giants? “Anyone taking this line has got an awful lot of explaining to do” (p. 1).

Paley (2002) has also suggested that critiques of “Cartesian” can be interpreted as a kind of psychological projection, or what he refers to as “displacement.” It is argued that most people who decry Cartesian dualism, on close examinations of their views, seem to be radical dualists themselves. Worse, their dualism is sometimes more extreme, and in some cases diametrically opposed, than the dualism put forth by Descartes himself (p. 1). Also, there is significant confusion on philosophical doctrine. “When nurses attack ‘Cartesian dualism’, what they are really attacking is materialism,” the view that human beings are nothing but “slabs of meat.” Paley rightly goes on to describe how Descartes the writer, the dualist, would have emphatically agreed with the nurses on this point (p. 2).

However, beyond this, Paley (2002) notes there is a “double irony” when examined further. Nurses who lament the “Cartesian” model typically identify “mind” wholly with feelings, sensations, and emotions, a point to which Descartes would have well-reasoned objections to. But they are correct in noting that he attempted a physiological explanation for these things, but this is something that nursing would agree with (p. 3). Paley thus opens up an immense amount of intriguing questions, to which only a few he attempts even tentative answers. How can we hold this immense complex of ideas? This is a question I would like to leave open for the moment, as it relates centrally to my overall research problem. For now, it is sufficient to note that several philosophers writing today are not only keenly aware of the divergence but are beginning to account for it as some kind of a psychological dynamism, a reality of its own. However, before leaving the philosophers, one work in this category merits a more detailed discussion.

Descartes' dualism

Of all the works cited in this study, one in particular plays a pivotal role, and so it requires a certain emphasis. This is *Descartes' Dualism*, by Gordon Baker and Katherine J. Morris (2002), professors of philosophy at Oxford. As mentioned earlier, this book played a pivotal role in my own exploration of the subject. Although originally published in 1996, it has recently gained in popularity, which supports the progression of awareness, as sketched above (Morris, personal communication, December 11, 2016). Overall, in terms of its concern for the overall problem, it includes elements of all categories mentioned above. However, this text is remarkable because of the focus and rigor of its central argument, which is central to my research.

Ever since Descartes' first published work, scholars have carefully debated the relative veracity of the various Cartesian doctrines, including of course dualism. Every truth claim that has ever fallen under this rubric has been rigorously studied, debated, dissected, and deconstructed. Baker and Morris (2002) feel that this has mostly been done competently (p. 2). However, the one truth claim that has curiously gone unnoticed, and therefore unexamined, is that Descartes was a Cartesian Dualist.

Baker and Morris (2002) question this assumption, thoughtfully and carefully. Based on close textual analysis, and using a philosophical hermeneutic lens, they present a very compelling argument that Descartes simply could not have been a Cartesian Dualist (p. 2). The first part of the book presents the argument, and the second provides a new interpretation of Descartes' dualism, following closely the source texts. For the purpose of this review, I will focus only on the first part. This is because at this point, I am less interested in what Descartes actually wrote than I am in what caused the misunderstanding in the first place.

In the preface to the book, Baker and Morris (2002) note an event from art history, in which a similar phenomenon can be seen. Briefly, a Dürer woodcut of a rhinoceros is noted by a critic to be a gross distortion of the real animal. The same critic prefers another engraving, termed "from the life," but this one turns out to have some of the same distortions (p. x). The point is that there may be a widespread human tendency to see "reality" not as objectively as we think, but rather with many of our own unexamined prejudices, and that such a tendency has a strong persistence because we want them to be true. Apropos, the authors include a prefacing quote from Wittgenstein, which suggests that the real problem we face is not that of the intellect, but of the will (p. v).

The legend

Baker and Morris (2002) refer to the common understanding of Cartesian dualism as the *Legend*, particularly insofar as it unquestioningly assumes that it, and it alone, is the correct interpretation of the source texts (p. 23). Interestingly, the authors employ this term almost in the third person, as if it were a little personality. Examples include: "The Legend has taught us all that . . ." (p. 4), "the Legend certainly never challenges this . . ." (p. 18), and "does the Legend seriously want to take passage (1) to argue that . . ." (p. 35). Again, whether the authors are aware of it or not, they are speaking in terms very familiar to cultural complex theory, and to Jungian psychology generally. In this tradition, the human psyche is envisaged as comprising a number of relatively autonomous sub-personalities, and these can function as quasi-conscious subjects in their own right. It is also noteworthy that they capitalize the word "Legend," as I do with "Split." For now, it suffices to say that Baker and Morris's Legend can be seen as an autonomous psychological force, which seems to yield a simplistic, yet naïve, interpretation of Cartesian ideas, and of their role in philosophic history. Further, like a complex, it perseveres. In spite of numerous criticisms, and of problems created by it, it "exhibits remarkable powers of recuperating from severe injury; indeed, it seems able to regenerate amputated limbs" (Baker & Morris, 2002, p. 1).

It is also noteworthy that Baker and Morris (2002) choose the word "Legend," and not "myth," as Ryle does. This is because they are concerned about a "second-order myth, a myth about a myth" (p. 1). Again, Ryle sees the Two Worlds view as a myth, denoting that it is not true as a model, but that it is true that it came from Descartes. Baker and Morris argue that even the second claim is not true, hence a "second-order myth." But because mythic forces have taken over an historical figure, they appropriately use the word "Legend" (p. 2). This is an appropriate use of terms, but for me, such "mythic forces" can refer to something that is both false and true at the same time. In other words, I agree with Baker and Morris that it is not true that Cartesian dualism came from Descartes, but, at the same time, I claim that it is true that something else, something unconscious, is making us believe it. Perhaps the word "myth," as I use it here, can describe this dynamism more effectively.

However, before proceeding with the content of their Legend, it is necessary first to define its scope. Consistent with cultural complex theory, Baker and Morris's (2002) define their culture, which is their community of academic philosophers (p. x), in a manner also similar to Cottingham (1998b, p. 19). Thus, their target audience is those who are intimately familiar with the primary texts, and generally all subscribe to the Rylean Two Worlds view. However, my target audience is somewhat distanced from this philosophic tradition, and have formed many other kinds of "Legends" in their own right, as detailed in the previous chapters. However, Baker and Morris's treatment must still be given special consideration because its source texts, such as Ryle, must have surely informed the other academic fields, from which all the other legends and myths were created.

The two worlds view

In this sense, it is useful to re-orient ourselves with the Two Worlds view and explore its implications in more depth. Again, this is essentially Ryle's understanding of Cartesian dualism and is aptly envisaged as the Ghost in the Machine. Although this view has been rigorously challenged, it at least has the benefit of being able to be clearly articulated and is internally consistent. This is not the case with the more extreme legends that have been superimposed on top of it, such as those found outside of philosophy, as in Capra. These are Radical Dualism, in which the two worlds never interact, and its apparent corollaries of Cartesian Materialism and Solipsism.

"Two Worlds" is certainly a beguiling image, particularly when framed with the frequently used antecedents "Inner" and "Outer." However, on inspection, there are immediate problems with these terms, both historically and semiotically. First, Descartes did not employ such terms, but we assume he did, or at least we assume he imagined them in the same way we do. Second, what kind of associations do we now make to the terms associated with the Outer World, such as "clockwork" and "machines?" And how have the meanings and associations we make to these terms changed over time, and across multiple translations? These questions alone should give pause to the attribution of any single interpretation to any one person, especially to a French philosopher who lived four centuries ago. And yet, the Legend still insists that Descartes was a Cartesian Dualist, in these terms already defined. To further highlight this problem, Baker and Morris introduce a few more terms and examples from modern philosophy, which helps to clarify how this understanding has developed.

First, how exactly should we translate the Latin term *cogitatio,* which figures so prominently in Descartes' writings, particularly his famous maxim "*Cogito ergo sum*"? This is a fine example, because it would seem straightforward, but turns out to be very difficult upon examination, as I have already previewed with Capra and Hillman.

Baker and Morris (2002) argue that the Legend interprets *cogitatio* as all possible states of consciousness, not just thought, but also sensations and emotions. Also, these states are frequently discussed in terms of their non-cognitive aspects (pp. 13–14). More critically, Descartes is understood to have innovated this usage. He is understood to have "broke with the medieval tradition," to expand the realm of mind (p. 15), creating a new category of mental entities, such as "sense-data" (p. 16). The authors refer to this as the Expansion Thesis (p. 14), and this amounts to the creation of a new world, the Inner World. This largely informs the justification of referring to Descartes as the "founder of modern philosophy" (p. 16).

Because thought is now *equated* with consciousness, in all its forms, this has necessary implications for the other world of the Two Worlds view. By definition, the world of physical objects, of things extended in space, must necessarily be devoid of consciousness. Therefore, the Expansion Thesis, as so defined, must always be accompanied by the Contraction Thesis, by which all physical objects, such as the body and animals, are "nothing but" unconscious clockwork. The result is of course the perceived deep split between mind and body, or between "consciousness and clockwork." Again, Descartes is credited with this as a radical innovation (Baker & Morris, 2002, p. 17). However, Baker and Morris agree with Ariew that Descartes's actual philosophy is much more traditional than is popularly thought (p. 63).

Now that the two worlds are more clearly understood, particularly in terms of the shift in the location of consciousness, the Legend then develops an understanding of the particular ways by which objects in each world are perceived and judged to be true. Curiously, the Two Worlds view here shows a strange mix of both opposites and similarity. The two worlds are polar opposites in terms of privacy, mode of perception, and fallibility. To illustrate this, Baker and Morris (2002) employ the thought "I am in pain" as an example. This thought is essentially private, only the "I" experiences it directly. Others can only indirectly infer it to be true. This has been brought under the heading of first-person and third-person asymmetry. Also, this thought is known only via introspection, which is a nonphysical faculty. Lastly, this process is "essentially and universally infallible" (pp. 18–19). In other words, the "I" may not know what is causing the pain, but it cannot doubt whatsoever that the experience of pain is happening. Thus, experiences in the Inner World are private, immaterial, and infallible.

By contrast, the Outer World is experienced in exactly the opposite way. Events are public rather than private. They are known only through the five external, physical senses, instead of the inner sense of introspection. Finally, these physical senses are fallible rather than infallible. Conspicuously missing from this entire characterization is the location and function of judgment, which is surely needed in both worlds, and also the process by which one comes to know one's own body (Baker & Morris, 2002, p. 28). In other words, judgment cannot be so easily located in either world, so it tends to be ignored.

However, in spite of these polar opposites, the Legend understands the processes by which the faculties operate to be of equivalent form. In other words, just as the Outer World is inhabited by physical objects with physical properties, the Inner World is inhabited by their counterparts: Mental objects with mental properties. The five senses perceive the former, while introspection perceives the latter, but both in a parallel manner to each other (Baker & Morris, 2002, p. 26). This is the category error as proposed by Ryle (1966).

The final component of the Two Worlds view is the supposed manner of interaction. According to the Legend, Descartes firmly believed in a two-way causal interaction between the two worlds. A physical event, such as light hitting the eye, causes the mind to perceive light. In a corresponding manner, the mind can cause the body to move, by first thinking the thought of motion (Baker & Morris, 2002, p. 21). As such, a human individual is seen as "'glued' together" by causal interaction (p. 27). This schema has been the subject of lively debates and is famously referred to as "Cartesian Interactionism" (p. 21).

In summary, the Legend, as presented by Baker and Morris (2002), defines Cartesian dualism as the belief in these two independent but parallel worlds. These worlds have their own inhabitants, of equivalent but opposite form. The Inner World consists of all mental objects, including all states of consciousness, and the Outer World of extended objects. Perceiving these two worlds is performed by opposite faculties, with opposite characteristics, but by similar process. Finally, the two worlds interact via two-way causation. It should be noted that the vast majority of modern philosophers have wide-ranging and contentious objections to this conception of reality but, at the same time, nearly unanimously agree that Descartes is the single, innovative source of it in the Western psyche.

Critiquing the legend

It is against this latter claim that Baker and Morris (2002) bring most of their arguments. I cannot possibly summarize all of these here; they are too numerous, detailed, and well researched. For now, I will have to rely on their own voice to summarize their conclusions from these arguments: "We argue that there is no solid *textual* foundation whatever for ascribing *any* single element of Cartesian Dualism to Descartes. On the contrary, many of the Legend's exhibits provide at least *prima facie counter*-evidence" (p. 23). In other words, some of the arguments used in support of the Legend contain elements that simultaneously refute it. Thus, there are likely widespread unconscious forces at work, which would explain why these exhibits have been so strongly mishandled.

Again, I admit to having been convinced, on the basis of these arguments, that Descartes was not a Cartesian Dualist, as the term is now understood. Any reader who is unconvinced, or wishes to examine these arguments themselves, is highly encouraged to do so. Even if Baker and Morris's arguments are not entirely convincing, the reader will benefit greatly from considering them thoughtfully. However, given the central importance of the Two Worlds view, it is worth examining a few of Baker and Morris's specific arguments.

The first argument I would like to highlight regards the aforementioned split between consciousness and clockwork. Recall that the Legend regards sensory perceptions as states of consciousness, and therefore must be part of the inner world, and so lacking in the mere "clockwork" of animals. This notion does have at least a partial basis in Descartes' writings. Descartes defines a thinking thing as "a thing that doubts, understands, affirms, denies, is willing, is unwilling, and also imagines and has sensory perceptions" (as cited in Baker & Morris, 2002, p. 31). Sensory perceptions, in the Aristotelian tradition, were governed by what was called the sensitive soul, which was a part of nature. Therefore many commentators have interpretated Descartes definition as effectively "shearing" off the faculty of sensation, or "extracting" it from nature, and thereby claiming it wholesale for mind. This is necessary for the Contraction Thesis.

However, a closer reading of the text yields some problems. Immediately after the above definition, Descartes devotes attention to *sentire*, or sensation, which comes up so frequently in context of the *cogito*. He distinguishes between a sensory perception proper and having a sensory perception.

It is only in this latter sense that he includes *sentire* as a thinking thing (Baker & Morris, 2002, p. 32). In other texts, he makes a similar distinction, this time using the specific examples of the perceptions "I am seeing" and "I am walking" (p. 31). For Descartes, these phrases qualify as thoughts only "in so far as we have awareness of it" (as cited in Baker & Morris, 2002, p. 31). Yet the Legend maintains that the entirety of these perceptions are "inner" things. If this were taken to its logical conclusion, then Descartes would have regarded animals as not having sensory perceptions at all. In other words, if "I am seeing" is an inner event, then animals do not "really" see; they are machines only. Commentators have stated, even explicitly, that this is what Descartes necessarily implied. But the original text clearly used the examples "I am seeing" and "I am walking" in an exactly parallel form. Therefore, the Legend would have to reason that Descartes would have also implied that animals do not "really" walk. This line of reasoning yields a *reductio ad absurdum* (p. 35). One could draw two conclusions: Either "the father of modern philosophy" argued in absurdities, or, our interpretation of his writings is absurd, or perhaps some of both. Unfortunately, most draw the former conclusion unilaterally, which, in my opinion, is more absurd than the latter.

It should be noted here that this argument may seem to run against several I made earlier. Critiquing the Legend in this way, by excluding sensory perceptions proper from *cogito*, would seem to provide weight to defining it purely as the intellect only, as in Capra and Berman. However, earlier I argued against this interpretation, because it completely excludes bodily states, which is clearly not in line with Descartes' writings. In other words, prevailing interpretations of *cogito* seem to be split between that of a purely disembodied intellect on one hand, and all states of consciousness on the other. However, crucially, there is room for a middle interpretation. Baker and Morris (2002) argue that there is one aspect of *sentire* that can indeed be called thinking, *and this is essentially the "thought" of sensation.* Hence, Descartes appears to be *disambiguating* the term, rather than placing it firmly into any one category (p. 32). This point is crucial.

There is also a related problem with our understanding of the infamous *Bête-Machine* doctrine. This is in reference to Descartes' alleged belief that animals are "nothing but" clockwork, or machines, and therefore inferior. Baker and Morris (2002) note that Descartes uses these two terms in different ways, and both have drastically different connotations than those of today. First, in the 17th century, clockworks were objects of universal admiration (p. 37). However, Descartes, strangely enough, reserves even more admiration for what he will call "machines." Clocks, however elegant and impressive, are still made by man. By contrast, bodies and animals are much more impressive and awe-inspiring, because, in his view, these are made by the hands of God. As such, the "machinery" of bodies and animals, according to Descartes, are superior to even widely admired clockwork.

As such, bodies and animals are capable of "exhibiting more artistry than I could possibly ascribe to it" (as cited in Baker & Morris, 2002, p. 37). Clearly, the meaning of the word "machine" has therefore drastically shifted since Descartes' time. We project our own associations of the word machine backward in time at our own peril.

Another significant problem with the attribution of the *Bête-Machine* doctrine to Descartes rests on the sensation of pain. The Legend, according to the above, interprets the sensation of pain as a purely mental object. Therefore, Descartes must have regarded animals as unfeeling mechanisms. This makes sense given that the Legend is committed to a dualism of mirrored faculties: The mental world is perceived by introspection, and the physical world by the five external senses. The perception of pain is not performed by the traditional five senses, therefore, it must be a purely mental event. Unfortunately, such a straightforward dualism is achieved only by ignoring the significant amount of exposition that Descartes dedicated to the two *internal* senses, one of which included the perception of pain (Baker & Morris, 2002, p. 48). Descartes' two internal senses, which can be summarized generally as pain and emotions, are difficult to place in the Legendary Dualism, so the Legend prefers to ignore them altogether. "'Internal sense' never occurs in indices of books analysing Descartes thought" (p. 49). Further, textual analysis strongly suggests Descartes treated the internal senses similar to the external ones, which would place them primarily in the body, and therefore also in animals (p. 50). Baker and Morris are of the opinion that the tension created by the notion of internal senses must be "intolerable" for proponents of the Legend. Perhaps the tension is dealt with via "repression," by neglecting discussion of pain altogether. A further repression is required to ignore Descartes' explicit treatment of the internal senses as similar to external senses (pp. 49–50).

Finding truth in myth

In summary, there has been extensive amount of research into the nature of the overall Descartes Problem. It is also striking how much the language of this work resonates with cultural complex theory. However, none of the works cited approach the problem specifically with a dedicated psychological lens, and only a few manage to assign it a full sense of psychological reality. Also, the majority of the philosophers eventually use the problem as a device in order to provide some kind of new interpretation of Descartes. By contrast, I wish to provide an interpretation of the problem itself.

In other words, the existence of a gross mischaracterization of Descartes is now well accepted, at least in some circles, but the psychological mechanisms behind such a phenomenon have yet to be fully explored. Further, a specifically Jungian view seems most appropriate for this, given that words such as "Legend" and "myth" are so frequently invoked in the existing accounts.

As such, the Cartesian Myth needs to be studied in its proper, *archetypal* context, in order for its full nature to be revealed. This is what is missing from all prior treatments. Those in the prior chapters assume that Cartesianism came from René Descartes, and those in this chapter, assume it comes from regrettable misunderstanding. Both are misguided in attributing the cause of the trouble to something human, all-too-human. In my view, the larger-than-life figure who is usually portrayed needs to be seen as something very different than either. In short, it needs to be seen as larger-than-human. This has already been betrayed by the existing commentary I have documented. Again, this is a figure who poisons our thoughts from the nether world, who steals the soul from nature, and imprisons it in the brain, and who forces us to believe that we live in Two Separate Worlds, despite all our best efforts for re-integration. *This figure will not be affected by any intellectual deconstruction*, regardless of how well we read the source texts. Rather, this mythic figure needs a mythic background, in order to fully appreciate its etiology, its genealogy, perhaps even its teleology.

Even so, beyond whatever fruits this approach may provide, I view my work as potentially supplementing the work already started by the scholars in this chapter. The task of re-interpreting Descartes authentically for contemporary times is likely to be very productive. However, it would be beneficial, and perhaps even required, to have a proper account of the unconscious psychological forces that have precluded a proper interpretation in the first place. In other words, an appreciation of the archetypal level of the complex may eventually serve as a working guide, or initial orientation, to the philosopher's task.

References

Ariew, R. (1992). Descartes and scholasticism: The intellectual background to Descartes' thought. In J. Cottingham (Ed.), *The Cambridge companion to Descartes* (pp. 58–90). Cambridge, UK: Cambridge University Press.

Baker, G. P., & Morris, K. J. (2002). *Descartes' dualism*. London, UK: Routledge.

Bennett, J. (1998). Descartes' theory of modality. In J. Cottingham (Ed.), *Descartes* (pp. 160–185). Oxford, UK: Oxford University Press.

Bolton, R. (1999). Dualism and the philosophy of the soul. *Sacred Web, 4*. Retrieved from: http://www.sacredweb.com/online_articles/sw4_bolton.html

Bracken, H. M. (2002). *Descartes*. Oxford, UK: Oneworld.

Cottingham, J. (1992). Introduction. In J. Cottingham (Ed.), *The Cambridge companion to Descartes* (pp. 1–20). Cambridge, UK: Cambridge University Press.

Cottingham, J. (1998a). Descartes' treatment of animals. In J. Cottingham (Ed.), *Descartes* (pp. 225–233). Oxford, UK: Oxford University Press.

Cottingham, J. (1998b). Introduction. In J. Cottingham (Ed.), *Descartes* (pp. 1–27). Oxford, UK: Oxford University Press.

De Rosa, R. (2007). The myth of Cartesian qualia. *Pacific Philosophical Quarterly, 88*(2), 181–207. doi: 10.1111/j.1468-0114.2007.00286.x

Garber, D. (1998). Descartes' method and the role of experiment. In J. Cottingham (Ed.), *Descartes* (pp. 234–258). Oxford, UK: Oxford University Press.

Lee, K. (2013). *Reading Descartes otherwise: Blind, mad, dreamy, and bad.* New York, NY: Fordham University Press.

Markie, P. (1998). The cogito and its importance. In J. Cottingham (Ed.), *Descartes* (pp. 50–78). Oxford, UK: Oxford University Press.

Paley, J. (2002). The Cartesian melodrama in nursing. *Nursing Philosophy*, *3*, 189–192.

Rodis-Lewis, G. (1998). Descartes and the unity of the human being. In J. Cottingham (Ed.), *Descartes* (pp. 197–210). Oxford, UK: Oxford University Press.

Rorty, A. O. (1992). Descartes on thinking with the body. In J. Cottingham (Ed.), *The Cambridge companion to Descartes* (pp. 371–292). Cambridge, UK: Cambridge University Press.

Ryle, G. (1966). *The concept of mind.* London, UK: Hutchinson's.

Sorell, T. (2005). *Descartes reinvented.* Cambridge, UK: Cambridge University Press.

Wilson, M. D. (1998). The epistemological argument for mind-body distinctness. In J. Cottingham (Ed.), Descartes (pp. 186–196). Oxford, UK: Oxford University Press.

Chapter 5

Ancient memories

At this point in the therapy, Ash has realized that the story of Rand is just that, a story. And yet, it persists, and continues to cause all kinds of trouble. The story is stuck on an endless loop, like an annoying song that cannot be purged from the mind. But worse than a song, this story is telling all sorts of terrible things about reality, and so it colors the entirety of Ash's perception. Something else is needed. We need to understand why this particular story features such a strong grip.

The therapist knows that humans are story-telling creatures. Since time immemorial, we have told stories to each other, at the very least to pass the time. However, some stories are much larger than these. These are the great stories, the legends and the myths, which do not grip just one person, but can enthrall entire civilizations, and persist for centuries. This story is now seen as no longer that of a mere father, but of *Father*, the Great Father, the One who created the World. The therapist knows that humans have told this basic story many times before. It is then helpful to compare this story with other Great Fathers, in order to better understand what kind of psychological underpinnings are at play.

In a similar fashion, in the preceding chapters, I have hopefully shown how Descartes is no longer the father of modern philosophy, but the Father of the Modern Era. Overall, it is a myth, and yet this myth is not false; it is its own reality, in a psychological sense. In other words, regardless of anything factual in philosophical history, something deep in our psyches appears to be heavily invested in recounting the following story: At the beginning of the modern age, Descartes made a Radical Split, separating all of reality into two. By doing so, he created the Two Worlds, the Inner and the Outer, and these categories of experience have dominated Western philosophical discussion ever since. In this sense, Descartes is certainly our Creator. Although there are many other mythological motifs that appear in this story, many of which I have already presented, this is the basic structure of the myth.

At this point, I must clarify my terminology. Thus far, I have used the words *image*, *myth*, and *complex* to describe the Cartesian Split, somewhat interchangeably, but they should be differentiated. By *image*, I mean to emphasize the psychological reality of the Cartesian Split, primarily in an introductory fashion. That is, regardless of whether dualism is a flawed proposition, the image of the Cartesian Split, particularly as expressed by Percy, is real, and this must be focused on closely. By *complex*, I refer to how this subject is usually discussed, characterized by irrationality, persistence, distortion, exaggeration, and excessive emotion. There is also a sense of unwarranted confidence. By *myth*, I refer to what can be imagined as the driving force behind the complex, or its element, the archetypal core. This mythic layer springs forth from unconscious depths, which can be seen to be energizing the various complex-ridden arguments. It may also be anticipating a resolution to the problem.

In the previous chapters, I tried to uncover this mythic layer from the complex layer. Moving forward, within this emergent myth, there can be seen two different strands. The first is from the traditionally philosophic discussions, and the other from a much broader field. These differences can be expressed in terms of the nature, and value, of the two worlds, as well as their manner of interaction.

The first is that which has already been identified by Baker and Morris (2002), the Two Worlds view. Again, under this conception, Descartes innovated modern philosophy by marking out brand new terrain, the private inner world of immaterial things. This was a separate world from material things, mutually opposed, but related in form, and these worlds were linked by two-way causation. Although most philosophers deny the truth of such a dual conception of reality, they mostly agree that understanding it is foundational to modern philosophy, and therefore worth at least a respectful consideration. Even Ryle's heated polemics included some conciliatory notes. Although this overall interpretation is questionable, it at least can be seen how it relates to the source texts. For my purposes, I give this conception a different name. The name "Two Worlds" is too general, so I refer to it as the *Mirrored Worlds*; however, the content is the same.

In the second strand, the two worlds are constituted by a much wider range of pairs of opposites. Also, they are no longer linked by two-way causation, but radically separated and isolated from each other. On account of this radical separation, there rises the possibility of one world eclipsing the other, as in Cartesian Materialism and Solipsism. These ideas are generally incompatible with the source texts. Finally, in contrast to the Mirrored Worlds, it is generally implied that the idea is not worthy of respect, it is even dangerous, and therefore ought not to be studied seriously at all. Rather, it is incumbent on the responsible scholar to outright reject it or heroically transcend it. I refer to this overall schema, content, and judgment of it, as the *Split Worlds* myth.

As has already been suggested, it is likely that the Split Worlds myth arose within a larger audience, who were most likely informed by the prominent Mirrored Worlds interpretations in dedicated philosophy. Therefore, the Split Worlds can be seen as a kind of continuation of the Mirrored

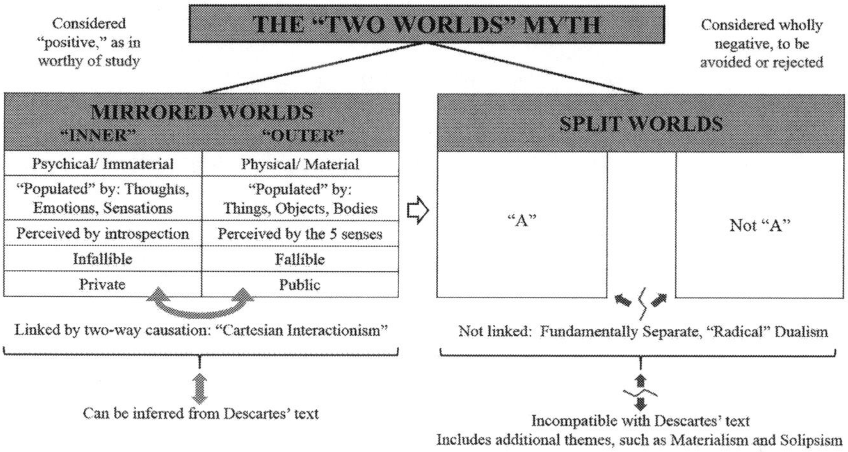

Figure 5.1 Summary of mythic elements.

Worlds. To assist in this overall organization of themes, I now include a diagrammatical summary of the above points.

Certainly, these two strands cover a very broad range of ideas across multiple disciplines, and therefore it may be risky to group them all under a single notion, the Cartesian Split complex, as I am attempting. It is difficult to imagine how these two strands share a common structure, particularly considering the magnitude of partial truths, distortions and emotional argument. However, perhaps it is on this very basis that they can be held together. In all cases, there are clearly mythic overtones, either by ridiculing Cartesian dualism as a myth or by describing aspects of it in overtly mythic terms. Therefore, I now turn to the world of myth proper, to seek out worthy material for comparison. In the Jungian tradition, this move is known as amplification, which seeks to identify a common mythic pattern or the underlying archetype. Each parallel by itself might seem tenuous, but taken together, the common pattern may emerge. I will start this process with the Mirrored Worlds and follow with the Split Worlds. In the following chapter, an interpretation of both will be offered, along with depth psychological lines, using the comparisons made in this chapter and following in the same general sequence.

Tales of the mirrored world

Upon reflection, the Mirrored Worlds myth appears to be a single species of a very prominent theme in comparative mythology, and this is the theme of the Underworld. There are innumerable instances in world mythologies which feature a land of the dead, spirit-world, or world of souls. This other world is beyond the conventional world, and yet coexistent with it. The two worlds are thus the day-world and the underworld. The latter is full of shadowy and strange forms that are similar to earthly forms, but at the same time, very different. The events in the underworld tend to obey a different set of laws or rules. The entrance to it, or threshold, is usually hidden or well-guarded. It usually requires a deed of some special ability to be able to cross the threshold. It is also usually a solitary experience.

Perhaps the best known example of this is the Greek underworld, or Hades. This world is marked off from the day world by the river Lethe, and guarded by Cerberus. Only a few have managed to journey to the underworld and return, such as Hercules, Orpheus, and Persephone, and these are solitary journeys. Although the occupants of the underworld are immaterial, being shades of the dead, each of these figures is able to interact with the living in a quasi-physical manner.

At first glance, it might seem a stretch to compare anything from philosophy to myth, but it is important to note that these traditions have intermingled from the very beginning. Plato concludes *The Republic* with the myth of Er, in which souls cross Lethe in order to be born, forgetting their other-worldly origins, the world of Forms. To remember these origins is the philosopher's task, and this must be done alone. A similar structure is found in the parable of the cave. In this tale, again, there are two worlds, separated by a threshold, and only one may break free to see the other world.

Perhaps an even better expression of the Two Worlds is found in Norse mythology, through the images of Asgard and Midgard. Asgard, the realm of the gods, is separated from Midgard, or Earth, by the rainbow bridge, another well-guarded threshold. Occasionally, a special figure crosses in either direction and interacts with the inhabitants of the other world in a manner similar to their own, even though they are of different natures.

The structure of the Two Worlds shows up in other traditions, and outside of conventional mythology. There is the generally well-known shaman's journey to the underworld and back, and the various vision quests of initiation rituals. These are also undertaken alone. Further, similar overall landscapes are readily found in the work of other prominent mythologists, such as Eliade's masterwork *The Sacred and the Profane*, in which the two worlds are in the title. It is also the backdrop for Joseph Campbell's (1973) famous monomyth, or hero's journey. One of the stages of this grand cycle is called literally the "Master of the Two Worlds" (p. 229).

It is crucial that the underworld is contained behind a threshold. In many cultures, the threshold is marked by a sacred place, or guarded over by specialists such as shamans, who have learned how to freely cross over the threshold at will. However, on certain days, such as the Celtic Samhain, the threshold is thinned, and so the dead can walk among the living. This naturally occurs shortly after the fall equinox, when the powers of light are balanced by the powers of dark, with the dark ascendant. Samhain is generally believed to be the ancient source behind our modern Halloween, a fantastic modern ritual literally showing us the Two Worlds. On this day, quasi-human figures are suddenly found walking the streets of ordinary neighborhoods, of course at dusk. Similar rituals are found in the Mexican Day of the Dead, among assuredly many others.

Closer to modern times, Jules Verne captured the public imagination in 1864, with his tale of a band of heroes who also cross such a threshold, the *Journey to the Center of the Earth,* which is of course a literal version of an "inner" world. In this tale, again, the inhabitants of the other world are very much Earth-like, but also very different. It is a prehistoric age, which might be Earth's early history, but at the same time, there are strange monsters and hints of a quasi-human civilization which may or may not be related to ours. Similar terrain was explored in many other classic science fiction stories, such as H. G. Wells's *War of the Worlds*, in which the other world invades ours, and *The Time Machine*, in which the other world is the future.

Many other "other-worlds" have thrived in our collective imagination. Alice tumbles down the rabbit hole to Wonderland, Peter Pan takes Wendy to Neverland, Dorothy gets whisked away to the Land of Oz, and Charlie ventures into the Chocolate Factory. These stories continue to exert intrigue, as all of these have contemporary re-imaginings in film and other media. The theme also finds new expressions. Currently, one of the most popular streaming shows is *Stranger Things*, which features a quasi-physical other dimension, parallel to our own world, but marked off by certain well-guarded thresholds, appropriately titled "The Upside Down." Finally, there are expressions outside of popular fiction. Perhaps we also physically incarnate these various stories at city fairs when we venture slowly through the spooky other-world of the Hall of Mirrors.

All of these classic myths and stories feature some notable parallels to the overall Mirrored Worlds myth. Recall that Ryle's inner world objects are opposite to those in the outer world, but still related in form, and are so are apprehended in an analogous manner, similar to the deeds in all examples above. In other words, the underworld figures of myth, being nonphysical, nonetheless share certain traits with things that are physical in nature. Another parallel is noted from the usually solitary nature of the journey, passing through a guarded threshold, whereas the events of the day-world are widespread and communal. This is essentially Ryle's notion of first-/third-person asymmetry, in which inner events are private, and outer events are public.

Again, it may seem spurious to suggest that detailed, critical commentary on philosophy has such analogues in myth. However, from a psychological perspective, it may make sense. Clearly there is an underlying pattern to all of these myths and classic, enduring stories. There is also a recurring human tendency to tell it in very different ways and in very different forms. Further, as I have already established, there are innumerable difficulties in understanding the "real" Descartes. Where uncertainties exist due to translation, cultural and linguistic changes over time, and dealing with obscure, difficult subjects to begin with, familiar tendencies can easily rush in from the depths to fill in the gaps, and restore lost confidence. It is also noteworthy that most commentators regard this conception of Cartesian philosophy with certain derision, regarding it as unsophisticated, or the province of "folk-psychology." Such an attitude might also be how they regard all of these childish "folk-tales."

Further, the parallels are not limited to just the Two Worlds themselves. Its attendant image, the Ghost in the Machine, also thrives in other forms. As before, the first instance of this Ghost may be from an ancient time, when myth and philosophy were combined. In various ancient Judaic texts, there are instructions on the construction of a Golem, a mechanical figure that can be infused with a spiritual essence, and become almost human. There is also the corresponding Neoplatonic doctrine of angelism, in which humans could be imagined as heavenly souls temporarily occupying an earthly body (Rodis-Lewis, 1998, pp. 201–202). In angelism, a soul could be imagined to remain, in essence, untainted by the sin of the body and its instinctual desires. However, the primary association of *Ghost* is that of a mysterious being from another realm.

This particular association has recently appeared, rather amusingly, in modern cinema. The 1997 film *Men in Black* featured a very small alien, of royal origin, who was found later to be operating a human-like machine from inside its head. Before this is revealed, the robot body was shown delighting in eating a meal. Interestingly, the entire film also employs a Two Worlds structure, in which the Men in Black are the guardians of the threshold, preventing the community at large from learning that there is another world in addition to this Earthly one. However, the singular hero of the movie crosses this threshold and learns the truth: That we are in fact coexisting with innumerable aliens, walking and talking among us, but they are all in disguise. Also, they are all generally anthropomorphic, but at the same time utterly different.

Another example of such a kind is the animated film *Inside Out*, in which each human character has a private inner world of various "ghosts," representing feelings. These characters operate the human personality by manipulating various bits of machinery, and these acts are hidden to other humans. The laws of this realm are similar to ours but slightly different. In other words, it is an exact portrayal of Ryle's interpretation. Although Ryle ridiculed it, it is worth noting that here it is at least a fertile ground for story-telling.

The Ghost in the Machine itself, or Golem archetype, appears prolifically in many other modern works of fiction. Generally, the theme is that a machine has been created which somehow acquires a special faculty, or the "ghost," which makes it virtually human, or in some case more than human. It becomes suddenly "self-aware." The earliest form of this is probably the classic tale of Pinocchio, a wooden puppet, who becomes alive and wants to become a real boy. This theme is echoed in films such as *A.I, Bicentennial Man, Chappie, Short Circuit,* and *I, Robot.* Other machines that develop human-like characteristics are found in *War Games, TRON, WALL-E*, and *She.* Sometimes the robots accompany human heroes and provide quality companionship, such as Data from Star Trek, the various droids of Star Wars, and the synthetic humans in the *Alien* films. In some cases, sentient robots become vastly superior to humans and become heroes themselves, such as in *Transformers*, the android Vision from the Marvel universe, *Robocop*, and the cyborg heroine in the appropriately titled *Ghost in the Shell.*

On the other hand, sometimes the development of the Ghost turns out horribly wrong. The first example of this is probably Frankenstein's monster, and the theme continues prominently today, with sometimes much worse outcomes. The machines become self-aware and turn against their human creators in the Terminator and Matrix films. Marvel's Vision was created to battle the self-aware villain robot Ultron. Similar tragedies are found in *Metropolis, 2001: A Space Odyssey, Blade Runner*, and with the Borg of Star Trek. This is the well-worn trope of the robot apocalypse, which is believed to be a literal truth by many, requiring real preparation. Even Stephen Hawking and Elon Musk have voiced their concerns on this. Others are more optimistic, such as Ray Kurzweil, who believes that the day of machine awakening will happen this century, an event he terms the Singularity. Not only does he believe it; he also insists it is inevitable. From this day forward, humans will be able to upload their consciousness into machines. Although losing our bodies will be somewhat tragic, the benefit will be becoming immortal, able to fly around the universe in self-replicating robot ships forever. This idea has inspired a movie of its own, *Transcendence.*

Overall, it is clear that the overall Mirrored Worlds motif is highly potent image, inspiring a vast array of modern folk tales. Either the two worlds are shown literally, or they manifest as the dual substances of the Ghost and the Machine. By themselves individually, ghosts and machines have been with us since the beginning of time, but when combined together, it forms a real marvel of imagination, both historically and in our modern times. As suggested, academics in philosophy, such as Ryle, are not immune to such a widespread and prolific image.

The first mirror

The Mirrored Worlds motif is also very prominent in various creation myths. These are especially relevant because the myth of the Cartesian Split is also a kind of creation myth, in the sense that Descartes is regarded as the "father" of modern philosophy, creating a radical Split in the known world, "in the beginning" of our modern age. First, it is worth noting that creation myths occupy a special place in the study of comparative folklore. Von Franz (1972) notes that whenever a creation myth is told by its followers, there is "always a certain *solemnity* that gives them a central importance." This is because creation myths ultimately concern the most important teachings, the origin of both ourselves, our problems, and of all existence (p. 5). It is perhaps for this reason that the word "radical" is often used, even though, as established, Descartes' philosophy is actually much closer to scholasticism than is commonly thought. The word *radical* comes from the Latin *radix,* which means "root," and this is certainly consistent with a creation myth. Von Franz (1972) also notes that creation myths are routinely told to the young, as a ritual of initiation into adulthood (p. 5). At this point it is worth pondering: Could it be that we have a modern incarnation of this same ritual today? After all, we commonly teach our undergraduates today by beginning Philosophy 101 with this most "radical," that is, *root* myth, that of the Cartesian Split.

Some version of the Two Worlds theme is found in almost every known creation myth. More generally, there is almost always some notion of two distinct substances being separated out from each other, from a prior state of unity, forming a pair of opposites, and thus the two worlds. A well-known example of this is found in the book of Genesis, on the very first day of creation. As the spirit moved over the waters in the Void, it said, "let there be light," and from this moment, light was divided from darkness, day from night, and morning from evening. In antiquity, the motif is found in perhaps its most general form, in terms of the root elements. For Empedocles, the entire cosmos is continually being created from the active presence of strife, or Neikos, which always strives to separate the elements into distinct substances.

The motif of creative separation is also found in many creation myths outside the Western tradition. In a Japanese myth, this comes in the form of personified substances, specifically the first world parents, Izanami and Izanagi. These two beings were originally in a state of union; however, the fates appeared to force them apart. Izanami died and was taken to the grisly underworld. Izanagi followed, but eventually fled in fear, placing a giant boulder between them, and they took an oath of divorce. In a fit of rage, Izanami promised to strangle 1000 people every day, but in return, Izanagi promised to help 1500 people be born (Hardacre, 2017, pp. 49–50). So ultimately, it was a constructive event. It was from this that the life and death cycle, which might imply conscious human existence, was first created.

Similarly, in an Egyptian creation myth, the sky goddess Nut was originally in a state of unity with the earth god Geb. However, from this state nothing ever happened, until Shu separated the two. Shu heroically raised Nut up, establishing her as the holder of the starry night sky. Frequently, Nut is graphically depicted in a dramatic overhead position, arching her back in a grand fashion to hold the sky up, allowing the many layers of creation to unfold underneath her (Pinch, 2004, p. 135).

This particular motif of the separated world parents finds its most dramatic expression in the Maori myth "The Sons of the Heaven and Earth," which is also a Mirrored Worlds theme. In this myth, again, the world parents originally lie together in unity and darkness, and so nothing happens. However, five of their children wanted to discover the difference between light and darkness, and so they conspired to separate them. The first four fail, because the parents do not want to be separated, and are very strong. But the fifth, Tane-Mahuta, finally succeeds. With a truly heroic effort, the hero's deed is what creates Heaven and Earth, and all of existence. It is only after this event that the people appeared (von Franz, 1972, pp. 156–157).

This myth is particularly noteworthy because of the wide variety of pairs of opposites being attributed to a single, creative event, similar to Genesis. Tane separates light from darkness, mother from father, Heaven from Earth, and day from night, all in a single act. This is very similar to the way the Mirrored Worlds are discussed. With one single book of *Meditations*, Descartes managed to separate inner from outer, mental from physical, subject from object, private from public, and certain from uncertain, thereby establishing the entire agenda of the modern world.

Other parallels may be noted. As was the case with Ryle, Descartes insists on an ongoing two-way interaction between the two worlds, in a manner similar to Izanami and Izanagi. Also, it is interesting to note that there is a long line of Maori heroes, who all fail, except for the fifth, and Tane only succeeds by trying a different approach. This could be related to the theme of the Heroic and Tragic Transcenders, only in this case, the heroes are attempting to split, and not unify. Finally, each of these myths are regarded positively because the division into two was necessary for creation, as is the case with philosophy students having to learn Descartes first.

In summary so far, the myth of the Mirrored Worlds can indeed be seen as a modern retelling of a very ancient story. In this view, the inner and outer worlds are just another incarnation of the day-world and underworld, and the Ghost in the Machine is yet another Golem. However, this myth is also a creation myth, accounting for the manner by which the two worlds were first separated, and also how they interact. The myths also show that the separation occurs between basic elements, or first parents, indicating that the separation is primordial, or pre-existing to all other human processes, and thereby positive. In general, all of these notions can be meaningfully compared to the Mirrored Worlds motif.

The dark mirror

However, the broader form of the Cartesian Split myth clearly has features that are not found in these myths, and these must be taken into account.

These elements move more toward the Split Worlds myth, in which the tone of conversation changes dramatically, regarding the value of the original separation. Essentially, the evaluation moves from that of a generally positive development to a more negative one, or one of creativity to something harmful.

This unique tone, of negative separation between two worlds, may be presaged in the Maori myth. This myth uniquely features a rather violent tone in describing the separation, bordering on the traumatic. Tane does not just separate, he "tore them asunder." Also, the existing powers resist: "Then wailed the heavens and exclaimed the earth—'Wherefore this murder? Why this great sin? Why destroy us? Why separate us?'" (as cited in von Franz, 1972, p. 157). However, Tane, the bold hero, disregards such complaints and pushes on to create the world and all the people. Also, it is noted that there was one child who did not conspire to join in the splitting, but five who did. This indicates that for the Maori culture at the time of this myth, the need for separation far outweighed the desire to remain united, and so this is still a positive separation.

Other creation myths also present a negative, more traumatic aspect to the act of separation. Even as far back as Empedocles, there is a rather dark tone assigned to this act. From the continually active strife of Neikos, there results sometimes unpleasant scenes of dismembered body parts and grotesque re-combinations. This calls to mind some of the emotionally charged images found in the source material, such as the Cartesian severed head, and Percy's "self ripped from self," resulting in chimeric monsters.

In a New Hebrides myth, there is a similar notion of violence, in that the land and sky do not wish to be sundered. However, the heroes push on and sing gleefully, "slice it apart. . . burst it apart. . . tear it apart," even as the sky and earth continue to groan and complain (von Franz, 1972, p. 153). Perhaps the most striking example of this is found in the Babylonian creation myth. Apsu and Tiamat are the world parents who lie together, and from this original state, again, there is no creation. The hero Marduk creates the world, but only after a prolonged and bloody battle. Further, Marduk does not just split the parents, but splits the mother Tiamet herself, by shooting an arrow down her throat. From Tiamet's dismembered body, the new world was created. One can see in this myth strong undertones of Bordo's characterization, in which the "organic female universe" was violently torn apart by a radical new world, the rationalistic modern era of Cartesian metaphysics, thereby separating itself from the Mother.

In summary, these particular myths include moderately traumatic aspects which lend themselves more closely to the Split Worlds motif. Overall, there is the sense of a primordial unity becoming tragically and painfully lost, even if the splitting was necessary. However, the Split Worlds features several other unique features that require further comparisons with other myths.

One of these is in how the central figure is regarded in terms of cultural impact. In the Mirrored Worlds, as I showed with Ryle, Descartes is seen as a worthy contributor to culture and the history of ideas, even if tragically flawed. It is often stated that his method was brilliant, but his conclusions absurd. Most also appreciate his style of careful reasoning, which of course even his harshest critics employ. In general, Descartes is seen as a human being, who at least gave a valiant effort in the pursuit of truth, and made significant progress toward displacing some of the centuries-old superstitions of the Dark Age. In these ways, Descartes shares a similarity with the heroes of the more positive myths studied thus far. In these positive creation myths, the one performing the original separation is a culture-hero for humans, and the ones being split are some kind of larger or older deity.

By contrast, in the Split Worlds myth, the Legendary Descartes no longer resembles a human, or a culture-hero for humans, in any sense. Rather, he is portrayed himself as a deity, almost demonic or anti-human, from a bygone era. Also, it is now no longer deities who are separated, but rather, it is the modern world of *humans* that is now radically and traumatically split, *by the deity*. The general mood is that, from this original event, nothing good has come, and therefore has to be undone in some way. As such, other mythological sources are needed to more precisely amplify these unique overtones of the Split Worlds myth.

A myth of this unique kind can be found, in germ form, in Aristophanes's speech in Plato's *Symposium*. The context here is a discussion on the origin of love, and an explanation is given by way of a myth. In this story, humans originally were round and consisted of two beings in one, facing opposite directions. One particular race, the Children of the Moon, embodied an original unity of opposites. They were both male and female, and were a kind of middle race, between the Children of the Earth and the Children of the Sun, because the moon shares in the nature of both Earth and Sun. These beings became powerful and too close to the gods. This angered Zeus, and so he split them down the middle, creating male and female. However, not content with this one violent act, he warned that if they ever acted up again, he would split them again, such that they would all have to hop around on one leg (Plato, 1952a, p. 157). Love therefore results from the pain of remembering our original unity, and our attempts to reunify, to undo the separation. Again, from this single act, as in many of the creation myths, we get many pairs of opposites: Love from pain, male from female, front from back, subject from object, and potentially left from right. However, even in this case of shocking violence, the act is still generally discussed in positive terms, or at least partially redemptive, as it is the origin of human love. There is also still the very real sense of a hope for reconciliation, as the beings can and do find each other, and restore unity. This hope, or driving force toward reconciliation, also implies a certain form of mutual interaction. The Split Worlds myth is therefore still quite different.

The original split

There is one other myth in particular that has all of the elements mentioned above, while also featuring a deity splitting human affairs, and almost entirely held in negative terms. This is the myth of the divided and flawed cosmos of Gnosticism, ruled over by the terrible and hated demiurge, the source of all evil in the world. This myth is quite unique in world mythology and offers many compelling parallels to the Cartesian myth. However, there are several difficulties in working with such material that need to be discussed first.

One such difficulty is its relative newness. Although the presence of the Gnostic myth has been known for millennia, it is only in the past few decades that a complete set of original material has been readily available, and scholars are still developing new translations and interpretations of it. I am referring specifically to the Nag Hammadi library, a recently discovered selection of 13 different codices, originally written in Coptic, and likely dated to the first few centuries of the common era. It is commonly assumed that these texts form a complete study library of some sort of Gnostic sect, or at least a group of people sympathetic to the unique tone and spirit of these writings. They were found, under rather dramatic circumstances, in a cave in present-day Egypt, and little else is known about who collected them. Before this material was available, there were only a few original documents available, along with generally unreliable second-hand critiques from the early Christian church fathers.

Another difficulty that has been raised by this ongoing evaluation is the complexity of the texts. Anyone even casually familiar with them will agree that the mythological motifs are presented in a bewildering variety of different names and images, along with several contradictions. It is now commonly understood that there really was no such thing as a single, cohesive group of people called "Gnostics." This is one of the more exciting and developing areas of biblical scholarship; the developing understanding that Christianity did not arise along clear dividing lines, orthodox and heretics, as the church fathers would have us believe. Rather, it is now readily apparent that there were many different groups and communities involved in the origins of Christianity. The texts of the Nag Hammadi library certainly reflect this kind of diversity.

As such, some scholars are seriously questioning if the label "Gnostic" should even be used anymore (Meyer & Pagels, 2007, p. 9). Their reasoning is that this umbrella term, which was not used by authors of the texts, but generally developed and used only secondarily by others, tends to marginalize these important differences contained within the texts. They also note that the term was used by the early church fathers in a rather pejorative fashion, who sought to label them as heretics, deviants from the one true faith. As suggested earlier, these accounts are usually taken suspiciously.

Overall, it is clear that the Nag Hammadi library, for all its riches, is not a single authoritative source text on "Gnostic myth," and so there is a risk of using it selectively and haphazardly.

For these reasons, I am assisted in my understanding of this subject by the work of Stephan Hoeller, who is the presiding bishop of a currently active Gnostic church, the *Ecclesia Gnostica* in America, and who has also written on Jungian topics. I have also studied Hans Jonas's (1972) *The Gnostic Religion*, one of the seminal works in the field. Each of these authors is keenly aware of the different traditions in the material, and yet would probably still maintain that there is still something that can be called Gnostic. If anything, I believe they would suggest, as I believe, that there is some kind of "Gnosticizing" tendency, active in the period of early Christianity, and that these texts uniquely exemplify this tendency. In any case, the selections I refer to for comparison tend to come mostly from the Sethian tradition, as well as some from the Valentinian works. Some have argued that the Valentinians were inspired by the Sethians, so I believe these selections constitute a kind set of mythological motifs that are relatively contiguous and consistent. Therefore, for the remainder of this work, by the term "Gnostic" or "Gnosticism," I generally mean Sethian-Valentinian. Finally, the material I draw from is a recently updated translation, edited by Marvin Meyer (2007), and which also includes helpful commentary, which aided my understanding.

The Gnostic two worlds

As presented earlier, the myth of the Two Worlds is very common in most mythological systems, and this remains the case with Gnosticism. This should not be surprising, as Jonas (1972) understands Gnosticism to be highly syncretic, that is, drawing on existing traditions. Specifically, Jonas argues that Gnosticism derives heavily from late Hellenistic systems, as well as from Jewish monotheism, Babylonian astrology, and Iranian dualism (p. 17). All of these systems can be seen to feature an overall Two Worlds cosmology, in terms of having a basic distinction between a mundane earthly realm and a supramundane heavenly realm. It seems that the Gnostics accepted this basic division of reality as self-evident, although I believe they developed this idea in many unique and novel ways, as I will show.

However, before this is explored in detail, it is enough for now to note how the overall Gnostic cosmology is usually summarized. Jonas (1972) identifies four common features of the Gnosticism, and one of these is they all maintain "a radical *dualism* of realms of being—God and the world, spirit and matter, soul and body, light and darkness, good and evil, life and death," and that such polarization affected both humans and reality as a whole (pp. 31–32). Such a sentence could not be better suited for modern evaluations of Cartesian Dualism, right down the specific words, including "radical." It also features the familiar long list of a wide range of pairs of opposites, and this is omnipresent.

In the texts themselves, themes of duality and pairs of opposites are found throughout. The Sethian *Secret Book of John* is one of these, which I will be referring to throughout this section. This text consists in part of a dramatic retelling of existing creation myths, including that which is found in Genesis, and also of certain Hellenistic systems. Many believe that this text is the best example of a Gnostic creation myth.

In this account, the universe is accepted to consist of heaven and earth, in this case the seven heavenly spheres, above five levels of the more material "abyss" (Meyer, 2007, p. 116). When the time came for the creation of humans, the two realms shook. Then, the psychic, or soul parts of humans were created first, followed by the material parts, with the resultant human being a composite of the two (pp. 118–124). After the creation of humans, Eve is shown to have had two sons, who are later to be revealed as the same as Cain and Abel. These two dueling brothers aptly demonstrate the theme of opposites, from the very beginning. The opposites here are bear versus cat, just versus unjust, and higher elements over lower elements. This latter pair is presented as the ethereal elements of fire and wind, versus the denser elements of water and earth. All of these pairs are in addition to the more traditional understanding of Abel as the representative of heaven, with Cain as that of earth.

All of the elements of creation are thus subject to these "two rulers," who are also both presented as being deceitful. Interestingly, this account includes other common Two Worlds themes. The two levels are together presented as a place of ignorance, a "cave," which obviously evokes Plato's cave. Further, there is a "water of forgetfulness," which evokes the threshold river Lethe (Meyer, 2007, pp. 127–128). Also, in a later section, a hero proclaims victory over all existence, from having completed several trips to the underworld and back (pp. 131–132).

In another text of unknown origins, the author recapitulates a certain long view of history in similar, dualistic terms. In the very beginning, there was only water and spirit, or elementary substances. Then, there was the first great age, that of flesh and matter. It was characterized by giant bodies, long periods of time, and was completed by the great flood. The elements of this age would then be the dense elements, water and earth. Following this was the second age, that of the soul, although this one was smaller, or "trivial." It is characterized by various harmful emotions and "unjust judgments." The elements of this age would then be the ethereal fire and air, and fire is featured prominently in this second age (Meyer, 2007, pp. 395–397). Although not mentioned, these two prior ages correspond to the lordships of Cain and Abel, respectively. Also, similar to the first account, a hero is promised for a future age, one that will defeat the underworld (p. 397).

In another text, the author dedicates quite an effort to explain the nature of the psychic, or soul world. The world of flesh and blood is presumed, of course, but the author insists on the realities of this other world, that of authorities and spirits, and these spirits are also presented as full of harmful emotions (Meyer, 2007, pp. 191–198). Again, Cain and Abel are presented, and both in an unfavorable light, with Cain as the man of flesh, and Abel representing heaven (p. 194).

Another presentation of these themes is found in a Valentinian text, commonly titled *The Tripartite Tractate*. This text features another retelling of the story of creation from Genesis, but as is typical for this community, the author elaborates by going back farther, to a point in time before the spirit moved over the waters. In this account, there is a kind of pre-existing pattern or template, from which subsequent acts of creation derive. This pattern features two orders, a higher thinking one rising out of a lower material one, and from the beginning, they are locked in mutual strife (Meyer, 2007, pp. 76–79). In one section, it is said that they were "engulfed by forces and material substances" (p. 76). These two orders eventually become heaven and earth, or soul and body, respectively. Specifically, the former is named "'those on the right', 'psychical,' 'fires,' and the middle ones,'" while the latter is named "'those on the left,' 'material,' 'darkness', and 'the last ones.'" (Meyer, 2007, pp. 83–84). The psychical realm is characterized by thinking, speaking, and images, as well as a lust of dominion over matter. The material realm is characterized by limitation, and certain blind, biological drives, such as procreation (pp. 85–86). This characterization is notably similar to the two great ages mentioned above. Humans are noted to have inherited this fundamental division, being a "depository of those on the left and those on the right. . . and his sentiments are divided between each of the two substances" (p. 87). Thus, it is not surprising to read that Adam and Eve would eventually taste the fruit of the tree of knowledge, which, in this Gnostic version, is described as having a "double character" (p. 88). This is because it allows for the knowledge of these opposites, specifically good versus evil. It also results in the expulsion from heaven to earth, which is of course another separation of worlds.

Several of themes are presented yet again in a dedicated creation story, titled *On the Origin of the World*. First, again, there were the original elements of spirit and water. Then, in a dramatic turn of events, the water itself becomes divided. The "watery substance" was placed in one region, which becomes heaven, and the "dry substance" placed in another region, becoming earth (Meyer, 2007, p. 205). The rulers of these two levels exhibit various pairs of opposites, having both masculine and feminine names (p. 205), and both heaven and earth shook under their influence (p. 206). And as before, these rulers exhibit many harmful emotions (pp. 214–217). And once again, the offspring of Eve are presented as a pair of unfortunate pairs of opposites, this time referred to more prominently as "psychical Adam" and "earthly Adam." The offspring of these two patriarchs fill the earth, but "they were all in ignorance" (p. 215). Also, in another text, this ignorance seems to breed strife. Eternal conflict is noted "both among the angels and among humankind: between those on the right and those on the left, between those in heaven and those upon the earth, between the spiritual powers and the carnal ones, and the devil against God" (pp. 672–673).

These selections bear striking similarities to the Mirrored Worlds myth, in which there are many dualisms found throughout creation, presented in various oppositional terms. What is particularly interesting is how these accounts resemble closely the Rylean conception of Cartesian dualism, in which the immaterial world consists of not only thought but also emotions. Although it is not presented quite this starkly in the Gnostic texts, the psychical realm seems generally associated with emotions, in some cases symbolized by fire. The material world, by contrast, is presented in both cases in a more limited sense, being either that of extension only, or in a very mundane sense, in which nothing of any real consequence happens. Also, it is noted that many of these texts declare that the entire system of dual existence is in ignorance, or presented as deceitful, or leading to eternal difficulty, much as how critics of Cartesian dualism regard that entire system.

It is also quite interesting to note how often the term "substance" comes up in these ancient texts, in many more examples than cited above. This is of course quite relevant to the notorious *substance* dualism of Descartes. The parallel is extended in the sense that in both cases, there is a dual system of opposite substances, one immaterial and the other material, and yet somehow they interact in a material fashion. Naturally, this is the ever-present critique of substance dualism, but it is very interesting to see this exact kind of interaction in an ancient mythological system. Further, the word "substance" itself can be seen as having certain mythological overtones, even outside of philosophy. In our current culture, for example, we no longer have drug addiction but *substance abuse*. In response, authorities do not restrict certain chemicals, but rather *controlled substances*. Something about this word seems to carry additional, dramatic weight, and could be related to all the consternation over substance dualism.

Of course, it is highly doubtful if the Coptic word for substance means the same thing to the ancients as the English word does for us today, but the similarity can still be noted. However, crucially, the Gnostics recognized a third substance, a purely spiritual substance. The problem was that this substance was very rare, or so well hidden or neglected that it was virtually non-existent. This substance was a very small remnant of a much higher realm, higher than heaven, but was lost and forgotten. Generally, the texts suggest that only a very small minority of people can see the third, or all three at once. This can also be positively compared to prevailing interpretations of Descartes. Whereas most see only a rigid dualism, Cottingham

(1998), who is one of the more accomplished Cartesian scholars, represents a minority opinion, that of a trialistic interpretation. I will return to the nature of this third substance, and the realm of the pure spirit, in subsequent sections.

The chief archon

Although the Gnostics were clearly concerned about living in a dual cosmos, and the attendant problem of opposites, perhaps even more concern was given to the creator of such a cosmos. This is the first ruler, the chief archon, who presides over all known existence. He and his various angels in heaven are the exemplars of all the terrible thoughts and emotions that plague humanity, as well as ruling over the mundane material world. In short, the mythic Cartesian figure, who today lurks in modern textbooks, powerful yet reviled, champion of both dualism and materialism, can be seen as a modern incarnation of a mythological figure, the Gnostic demiurge.

The word "demiurge" likely begins, fittingly, with Plato as well. In the *Timaeus*, the creator is notably portrayed as significantly less than omnipotent, perhaps even demoted, to a role much more humble and relatable. Rather than a supreme, impeccable being, god becomes more of a well-intentioned and skilled craftsman. Thus, the name Plato uses derives from the Latin *demi-ourgos*, which roughly translates to "public worker." Also, the work of this creator was inherently limited because it could only be an imperfect incarnation of an ideal Form or pattern, from which it was derived. Finally, the creator does not even get credit for creating some of the patterns, for many of these were already in existence (Plato, 1952b; Zeyl, 2014, para. 1). In this sense, the Platonic creator and the resulting creation, although good, were certainly not perfect. As such, it is necessarily implied that there was more work to be done by the soul, upon arriving in this world. For Plato, this generally involved a process of learning and remembering the nature of the ideal Forms.

Clearly, the Gnostics were heavily inspired by Plato, taking up many of these themes. But they also took this idea of an imperfect world and an imperfect demiurge in a radically new direction. Far from a public worker doing the best that he could, the Gnostic demiurge is incompetent, or sometimes malevolent. The Gnostics took liberty with other sources as well, and one of their favorite stories to rewrite was the book of Genesis. Whereas the Judaic Yahweh divided heaven and earth and proclaimed that "it was good," the Gnostics strongly objected. For them, nothing of all known creation was good. Rather, creation was inherently flawed *because it came from a flawed creator.* From various texts, he is "wicked in the mindlessness within him" (Meyer, 2007, p. 116), "an arrogant beast" (p. 196) whose "thoughts were blind" (p. 191). Further, "the chief creator was a fool"

(p. 209), who "reigned over chaos and the underworld" (p. 726). He tried to create a good world, "but he failed and did not get what he hoped for" (p. 179). The parallels to Descartes here are self-evident.

Primarily, the Gnostic cosmos was understood to be flawed on account of the creator acting out of profound ignorance. Although certainly having "great authority" (Meyer, 2007, p. 204), the demiurge is also shown to be ignorant. Particularly, he is unaware that a vast structure of prior creation and higher gods preceded him, and this lack of knowledge results in all sorts of trouble. Also, he is ignorant of his divine consort, Sophia, who was with him in the beginning, but who later withdrew to higher spheres. Left all alone, this arrogant, blind god, usually named Yaldabaoth, performed the original act of creation, patterned after various prior acts of creation, but he is unaware of these. Seeing himself as all alone, he claims the result for himself. The result of this is the entirety of our known universe.

It is also quite clear that the hated demiurge is strongly associated with an original separation of elements, in the manner of other creation myths. After separating the watery substance from the earthly substance, he "created for himself a dwelling place and called it heaven, and from matter, he created a footstool and called it earth" (Meyer, 2007, p. 205). Similarly, "to each <of> the two orders. . . he gave a name" (p. 83). This is of course similar to how Descartes notoriously named the two substances, *res extensa* and *res cogitans*. Further, in both cases, the creator retires to the upper realm only, and despises the lower, although still exercising complete command over it. "Yaldabaoth assumed authority over matter" (p. 204). This is seen today in the "rationalist" Descartes, who distrusts matter and the senses, and yet somehow also becomes a master of mechanistic reduction, the laws of nature. And finally, of course, both events occurred "in the beginning," and both were performed by deviant "Fathers," who are somehow both foolish and powerful at the same time.

Also, in many of these various creation myths, the authors emphasize that demiurge did not even create the original substances. Actually, this notion is implied even in the orthodox Genesis, as the spirit moves over the waters, without any account for who created the waters. In the Gnostic texts, the original "watery substance" of creation is detailed to have preceded the demiurge (Meyer, 2007, p. 204), or it is implied in various other ways that matter is associated with the pre-existing Sophia (p. 196, 261). Thus, the demiurge's creative act appears to be limited only to the *separation* of substances. This can be compared to critics who consider Descartes to be entirely unoriginal, merely recapitulating Augustine. And again, in the Gnostic texts, the creative act is flawed not from the act itself, but only on account of performing the deed out of ignorance. This is also the same with Descartes. Dualism in general can be a defensible philosophical proposition, going back at least as far as Plato. It becomes repugnant only when Descartes makes the separation, and this is exposed along with descriptions of some kind of regrettable blunder or error that he committed, very similar to the Gnostic texts.

There are also general parallels with the nature of the demiurge and the others like him. These quasi-human figures, collectively referred to as archons, reside in heaven, yet can easily walk and interact with humans on earth. Thus, although they are immaterial, they are considered very much real. This point is taken up directly in the title of a classic text, *The Nature of the Rulers*, in which the word for "Nature" is sometimes translated as "Reality." This indicates the author is trying to convince someone that the invisible powers are indeed real (Meyer, 2007, p. 188). Further, as presaged above, Gnostics generally associated this realm not only with thoughts, but also emotions. All the horrible deeds of the archons are ultimately the expression of emotions, such as jealousy, anxiety, lust, and so on. And as such, they are usually described as having animal faces (p. 192). In this way, the nature of the immaterial beings are described in material terms, while still being that of an opposite, which is precisely how Ryle critiques *res cogitans*. Finally, although the archons control matter, it is clear that their essence is essentially psychic, or that of soul. This is demonstrated in a lengthy account of creation, in which the archons create images of material things, directly alongside various "mental" faculties, such as sensation, perception, imagination, will, and all the emotions (p. 119–124). This myth then is an exact parallel to what Baker and Morris have referred to as the expansion and contraction theses, in which emotions, combined with thinking, sensations, and the imagination, are wholly within the immaterial or psychic realm. In both cases, matter is usually portrayed as wholly passive. In the myth, matter simply follows the pattern of the psychic images, similar to how Cartesian matter is often described as being "nothing but" matter.

The demiurge has many other unique characteristics that have uncanny parallels to the Cartesian figure, and this goes back to the moment of birth. The demiurge is born imperfect and deficient, or "misshapen" (Meyer, 2007, p. 115). This is because he is formed out of the lowest dregs of matter, "like an aborted fetus" (p. 196, 204). Because of this, his mother "was in great sorrow and anguish" (Hoeller, 1989, p. 141), and subsequently departed, such that "he did not see her face" (Meyer, 2007, p. 204). Similarly, Descartes was born with a near fatal illness, and his mother died when he was an infant. These details of course come from the historical account, not the mythological. However, it seems that these facts are often repeated by critics to an unusually high degree, perhaps because the historical facts have mythic resonances. Another reason could be an attempt to try to explain his failed philosophy from his tragic upbringing. This may be with some merit, however, as Descartes did write that he considered his chronic poor health in adulthood as something he inherited from his mother. Interestingly, in the Gnostic myth as well, the demiurge constantly suffers from various "painful and destructive passions," because his world is born from the same experiences of his mother (Hoeller, 1989, p. 106). Of course, both the demiurge and the Legendary Descartes grow up to be very powerful, in spite of their sickly origins.

The birth of the demiurge was a traumatic event at all levels. In *The Tripartite Tractate*, a prototype of the demiurge, the Logos, himself "suffered a division and a turning away" after his birth, for acting out too hastily against the preceding order. From this came "the faltering and the division came oblivion and ignorance of oneself" (Meyer, 2007, p. 73). Such a description demonstrates a clear parallel to Bordo's (1987) understanding of Cartesian dualism. Although she generally avoids recounting Descartes' troubled relationship with his historical mother, she does present a mythical version of it, considering that she understands Cartesian dualism to be uniquely symptomatic of a traumatic separation from the prior "organic female universe," the "mother-world of the Middle Ages and Renaissance" (p. 5), and a "flight from the feminine" (p. 9). Further, for Bordo, this event has resulted in an altered, unnatural conception of the self (p. 4), and this can be compared to the well-documented ignorance of the demiurge.

One of the first acts of the demiurge after coming into being was to declare himself ruler, for "he thought that only he existed" (Meyer, 2007, p. 205). Here he matches Yahweh word for word, declaring, "I am God and there is no other God beside me" (p. 116). Further, the name Yaldabaoth itself derives from the Hebrew Yahweh, which means "I am that I am" (Hoeller, 1989, p. 148). This declaration appears in many other texts; the crucial difference for the Gnostics over the Judaic account is that this declaration demonstrated ignorance. Similarly, Descartes is famed, and mocked, for establishing his entire philosophy by denying every other possible reality except for his own existence. Also, although it does not seem to follow, this immaterial *cogito* is understood to allow for a continuous understanding of the material world. Descartes notoriously derives from his own thought the mathematical laws for the motion of all material things, which later became the laws of physics. In the Gnostic myth as well, the demiurge immediately "assumed authority over matter" (Meyer, 2007, p. 204).

Finally, the demiurge is described with physical attributes that are surprisingly similar to modern depictions of Descartes. In the Gnostic myth, he and the other archons are described as androgynous (Meyer, 2007, p. 192), and this can also be seen in the rather effeminate characteristics of Descartes in modern portrayals. Such androgyny can be seen best when compared to Newton, who is often portrayed as more heroic and masculine. Whereas Newton is often upright with a broad chest and chiseled features, Descartes is often seated, in his robe, with his stocking-legs sticking out lengthwise (see figure 5.2).

And yet, although the archons are androgynous, it is clear that they are still essentially masculine. In one text, they are documented in lurid detail, running about creation with explicitly phallic behavior (Meyer, 2007,

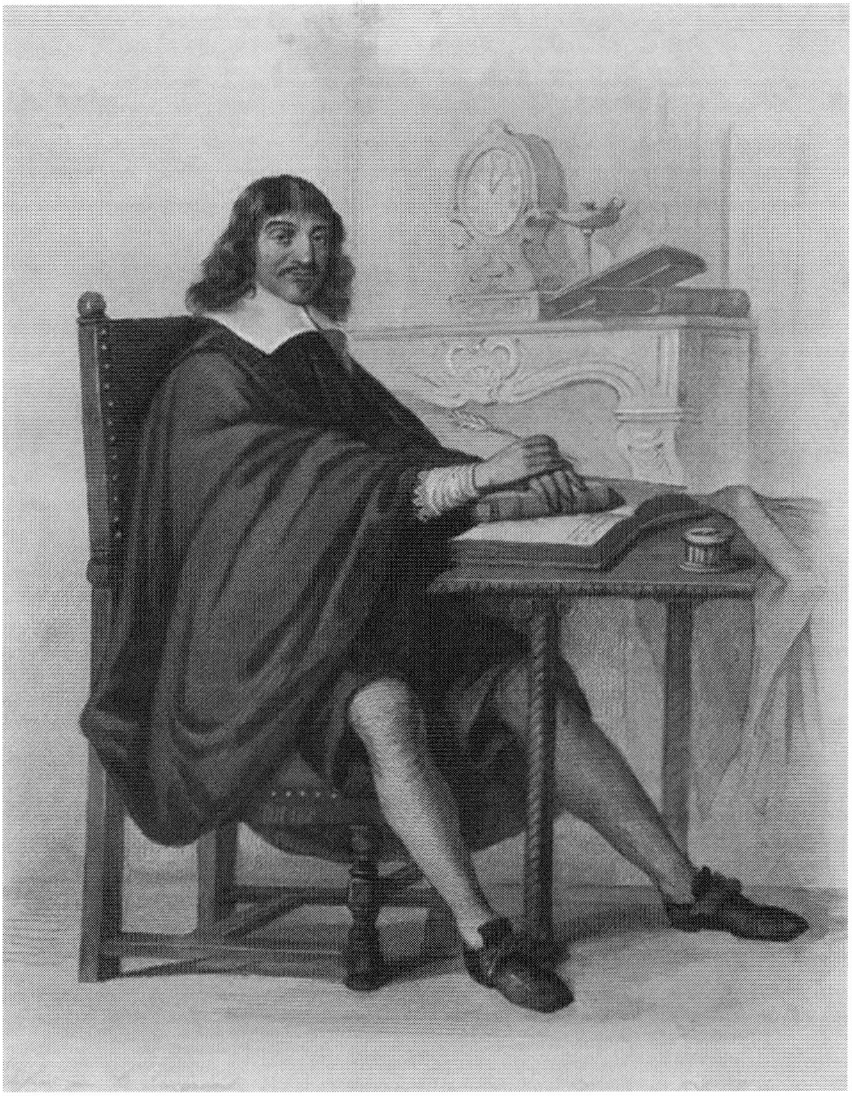

Figure 5.2 Descartes, by Baudran.

pp. 193–196). Similarly, we see Bordo (1987) take a sickly, effeminate figure, and at the same time, argue for a "Cartesian 'masculinization of thought,'" in the beginning of the modern era (pp. 8–9).

Descartes is also portrayed above with a rather dumb look on his face, as if he were a simpleton, easily confused. This is of course quite fitting, given

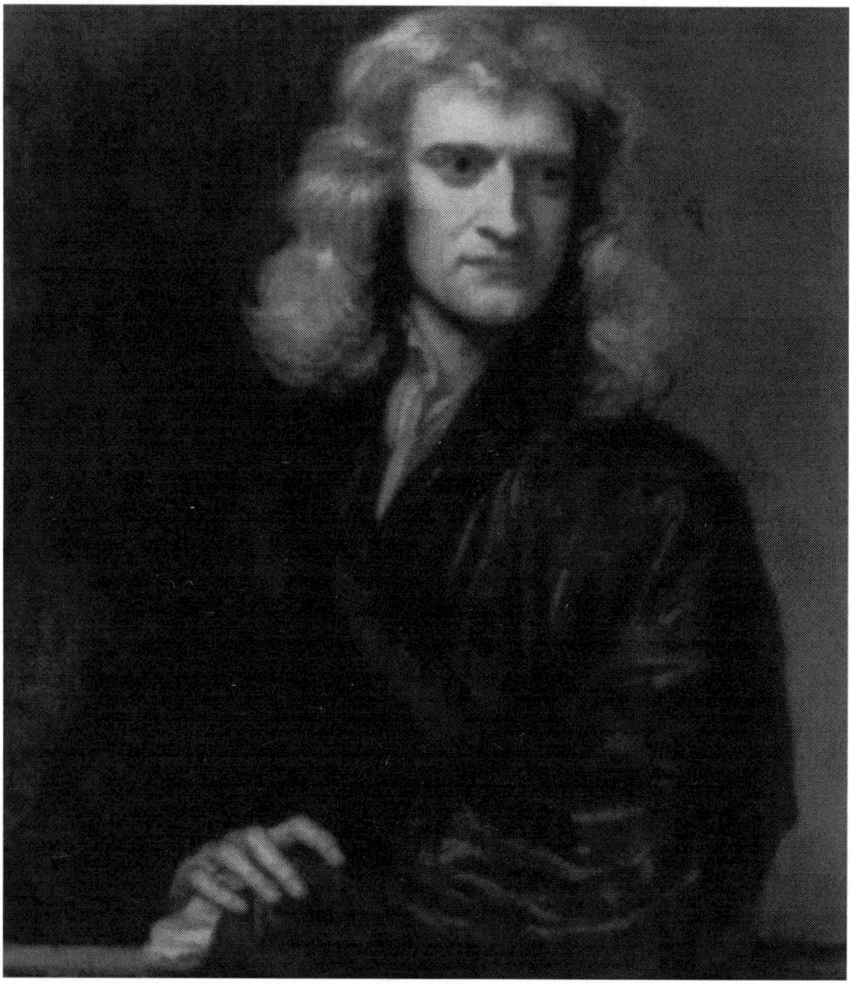

Figure 5.3 Newton, by Kneller.

how his philosophy is often criticized, and this is quite similar to the ignorance and foolishness of the demiurge. Also, the demiurge is described as having "the figure of a snake with the face of a lion" (Meyer, 2007, p. 115). The snake-like lower portion could explain the unusual prominence of the stocking-legs, which may be unique in portrayals of famous philosophers. Interestingly, in other versions of the same image, you only see one snake-like leg. Also, Descartes' facial hair and pronounced nose could certainly be described as lion-like. However, the most curious aspect of this and other prevailing depictions of Descartes is the sly grin on his face, and raised eyebrow, as if he is planning something devious. One could easily imagine him twirling his mustache, like the devious Captain Hook might, concocting another clever scheme to foil the heroes.

There are many other examples such as this. Earlier I compared Descartes' reputation to a viral meme, but in another way, he *is* a viral meme. There are an astonishing variety of curious depictions of Descartes floating around the internet today, much more so than comparable historical figures. The reader is encouraged to do a simple image search to see how many different ways Descartes lives on in our collective imagination. Many of these imply a mixture of maliciousness and stupidity, much like the demiurge. Also, many are heavily distorted, featuring wildly disproportionate features, showing almost literally the nature of a complex.

The splitting of the demiurge

When the demiurge "suffered a division," this may have had an unusual result. On one hand, he is depicted as a single being, believing himself to be alone at the beginning of creation, and also feeling the need to boastfully remind everyone that there are no other gods. On the other hand, he immediately creates an entire race of subservient gods, the archons, all made in his image. In some texts, they are there in the beginning, alongside the first ruler, without any reference to being created. These lower gods later play very prominent roles, in both further acts of creation, and in the everyday affairs of humans. From all this, it is sometimes difficult to distinguish between the activity of the chief archon and any of the others. It is as if the demiurge is both singular and multiple at the same time, with these two modes being almost interchangeable. Perhaps his very nature is inherently divisible or prone to splitting, and this is symptomatic of his ignorance or his traumatic birth.

This phenomenon is borne out in several interesting ways in the texts. "Yaldabaoth has many faces. . . so he could show whatever face he wanted when he was among the seraphim." Further, "in his thought he united the seven powers with the (archons) that were with him" (Meyer, 2007, p. 116). The interchangeability is also demonstrated with a curious usage of pronouns. In one instance, "he" tried to create a human, but in the very next sentence, "they" could not make him rise (p. 192). Also, the many are frequently portrayed in Gnostic myth in ways that are familiar to us from the canonical scriptures as the one. For one example, it is "they" who decide to make man, set up the garden of paradise, and issue the command to not eat from the tree of knowledge (pp. 192–193).

This interchangeability of the one and many also finds expression in the fact that the demiurge had multiple names. "This gloomy archon has three names: the first is Yaldabaoth, the second is Sakla, the third is Samael." The translators define these names as "child" or "child of chaos," "fool," and "blind god," respectively (Meyer, 2007, p. 116). The same run of three names is repeated in another, related text (p. 725). In another section, he is given a fourth name, "Ariael," because "he is like a lion" (p. 204). A fifth is "Nebro," which is interpreted in the text as "rebel" (p. 766). In this last text, "Sakla" is given to be a different angel.

This pattern has a strong parallel in the Split Worlds myth. Recall that for many authors, Descartes was singled out as both the primary influence on the modern era, while at the same time indiscriminately grouped with all other Enlightenment figures, a pattern I called the sub-Fathers. This was particularly evident with Capra, who described the progression from Galileo all the way through Einstein as a kind of fulfillment of a singular Cartesian vision. Similarly, for Hillman, Descartes was both the chief "arch-enemy," while at the same time just one of the four horsemen of the apocalypse. In other cases, it is recalled that the word "Cartesian" is frequently used interchangeably or in combination with others, while still having the same meaning, such as "Newtonian," "Cartesian-Newtonian," "Cartesian-Kantian," or the "Descartes-Locke-Kant tradition." These patterns often show up even for authors who still regard Descartes as the central figure. Also, in these cases, the words are used to describe a system of rules that is overall hindering or deceptive, or perhaps naïve, although still accepted by an unreflecting majority, just as the case in the Gnostic texts.

A terrible world order

After separating heaven and earth, the demiurge gets to work fashioning an elaborate and highly detailed kingdom in heaven. The authors of these texts seem to be fascinated by such intricate order, and at the same time, quite horrified by it, as we might be today with a stifling bureaucracy. In one text, the first act is the creation of 12 authorities, seven for heaven and five for the abyss, and each is individually named. Then, seven primary "physiques" are created, each corresponding to the days of the week. Then, as is typical for the archons, each is associated with an animal face. Each of these further subdivide, until the total number of angels is 365, one for each day of the year. Then, seven primary powers are created, related to the spheres of heaven, and named again. The text indicates that having two names is associated with a kind of cosmic, engulfing destruction (Meyer, 2007, pp. 115–117).

This dizzying hierarchy is then seemingly duplicated with the composition of what will become the first human (Meyer, 2007, pp. 119–124). Over the course of five pages, almost every conceivable part of the human prototype is carefully detailed, along with the name of its respective archon-creator. The precision is equally astonishing, for example, there is even a distinction between the teeth and the molars (p. 119). Also, many items in this list come in pairs of opposites, the right and left. The author dutifully notes that the entire composition, although impressive, is still to be regarded with deep suspicion. The primary elements are given as all-pervading "demons," and these demons produce all sorts of terrible emotions and feelings (p. 123–124). Again, the overall deficiency is not attributed to the quality of work, but by doing it out of ignorance. "He mated with the mindlessness in him," to create all this for himself (p. 115).

One can see in this myth a modern parallel, in terms of how academic philosophers regard Cartesian dualism. Those who have studied it in detail generally agree that it features an impressive set of well-reasoned arguments, with typical "Cartesian" clarity and precision, but also often argue that the entire system is flawed, on account of one singular and careless blunder. The blunder itself depends on the critic, but ranges from notions such as the Cartesian circle, a flawed reliance on the *cogito*, or his inability to distinguish between consciousness and self-consciousness. In the same way, the demiurge creates a dualistic, divided system that dominates the cosmos, just as Cartesian dualism has dominated the Western worldview, even though both are believed to be flawed on some fundamental level. This is common among both Mirrored Worlds and Split Worlds myths, although the degree to which the error is emphasized leads more to the Split Worlds.

The Gnostic demiurge delights in this creation of a highly systemized order of reality, in which everything would seem to fit together perfectly, with all details accounted for. This notion is beautifully depicted by Blake, who many believe to have strong Gnostic tendencies. In his painting *The Ancient of Days,* a demiurge-like being looks down over the created world holding a measuring device of some sort, similar to a compass. This could be compared to the image of a rationalist Descartes looking down on the world of extended things.

The system may fit together perfectly, but only at the expense of the people living within it. His lowly subjects are apt to quarrel endlessly about minutiae, in an arrogant and hostile manner. The "order was entangled in a struggle against itself," and "nobody agreed with anyone else about anything." Also, such followers assumed they were wise, but the Gnostics believed them all to be in error (Meyer, 2007, p. 89). However, the deficiency was not limited to general confusion. One text describes the prevailing world order as a place of perpetual bondage and enslavement (p. 86). This notion of the cosmos as a prison is perhaps one of the more distinctive notions of the Gnostic cosmology. The demiurge is flawed, but also very powerful, and this manifests in an unusually strong ability to keep humans enslaved, in the prevailing systems of both heaven and earth.

He also sets up these systems such that the people of the two orders continually flail against each other, in perpetual strife. Those of heaven, "the right," are destined to be distracted by materiality, and fall into sickness and evil, while those of earth, "the left," are destined to be ruled over by those with a "lust for dominion," which seems to be those of the right. Thus the entire system is locked in a negative pattern, where the worst of one side controls the other, and in between them is "fear and despair, oblivion, confusion, and ignorance" (Meyer, 2007, p. 83). Interestingly, this abject middle layer also serves as a kind of insurmountable barrier, a power that is "separating" those of the right and those of the left, preventing movement across. This is a classic Cartesian Split. Also, the demiurge is invested in keeping humans going in this two-world strife, because "they are useful for the economy" (p. 84). Later in the same text, the opposites are shown again in mutual strife, with "the right copying those on the left and those on the left also copying those on the right" (p. 88).

To ensure the status quo, the first ruler sets up a terrible hierarchy of authoritative rules, coercion, lies, and punishment. The existing order "should be kept in check" by such means, though a system of "commanders and subordinates in positions of dominion" (Meyer, 2007, p. 84). If humans get too wise, the archons make various devious plans to keep them in deception, preventing them from ever learning more about their condition. These "criminals" make a "phony spirit," to keep them in a "cave" of "forgetfulness" (p. 125). They promise a paradise, but "their pleasure is a trap, their trees are a sacrilege, their fruit is deadly poison, and their promise is death" (p. 126). They are also able to employ mind control, bringing "deep sleep," "drunkenness," and "making their minds sluggish" (pp. 126–127). They also try to scare humans to keep them in line, by giving them "a great fright" (p. 215). Punishment involves shortening their lifespans, and keeping what is left of them in "grief and weakness and evil distractions" (p. 217), or throwing them "into great confusion and a life of toil" (p. 194).

This system of devious enslavement is similar to the notion of perpetual Cartesian influence. For Capra, all major developments of modern science have been in service of fulfilling the Cartesian project, all the way through Einstein, even if this is against our better interests. This is the image of the Evil Genius, who, like the demiurge, plans traps for human minds in advance. Similarly, Frege compared residual Cartesian influence to a virulent boil, infecting all contemporary thought, much like the phony spirit polluting weak minds. Also, for Thomas (1996), the entire postmodern movement is still Cartesian, in spite of all its professed desire to be freed from it (p. 1). Finally, for Cottingham (1998), Descartes is truly the father of the modern age, because he set the agenda for all subsequent philosophical debates (pp. 1–2). Under this line of thought, no other thinker since then has had the freedom to even question the agenda, but rather, has been compelled to debate amongst each other within it. In other words, even those who claim to have outright rejected Cartesianism, cannot do so without implicitly accepting its agenda. It is indeed an all-pervading system of devious entrapment.

The first machine

The demiurge is portrayed as a foolish creator, and this is especially the case when it comes to the creation of humans. Prior to this, he and the other archons fashion the cosmos as they see fit, and things generally proceed according to plan. Then one day, something fundamentally different happens. The higher gods decide to project an image of a perfect human, a kind of spiritual prototype, or simply "Man" (Meyer, 2007, p. 118). The archons see this and are greatly impressed, and after much commotion, decide to try their hand at making a copy for themselves. However, the early attempts are lessons in futility. Perhaps it was known in advance, as Sophia laughs at their decision, knowing their ignorance. "They did not know what they were doing" (p. 212). Sure enough, their first creation "did not move or stir at all" (p. 124). They then try to animate it by breathing a soul into it, "but could not make him arise," and yet proceed to keep blowing, hoping for a different result (p. 192). In one account, this condition persists for 40 days, and the lifeless lump is called "an aborted fetus," much like the demiurge's own creation. Eventually, they manage to get Adam up and around, walking and talking, but there is still something lacking. Although he is body and soul, he is completely under the rulers' control. But with the help of Sophia, and sometimes the divine serpent along with Eve, he is able to gain true life, and become free for the first time (p. 125, 193, 214).

In these accounts, there are striking overtones of a familiar notion, that of the "notorious" Cartesian doctrine of the "*Bête-Machine*." Again, this is the view that human bodies, as well as animals *in toto*, are merely moving machines. They may be highly intricate, with the ability to move and speak, but they are lacking in some kind of critical, special essence. What is missing is what the Gnostic myth calls "Spirit," which is the third substance, beyond mere Body and Soul. Recall that when the archons formed the psychical body, this included all the things that we might find today in a highly sophisticated robot-machine, such as sensation, perception, and an "impulse to action" (Meyer, 2007, p. 119–124). But for the Gnostics and for us today, this is not enough. The machine at this point lacks its ghost, its true Spirit. In the modern version of this myth, this will occur at some miraculous moment in the future, the Singularity, when the machine finally achieves full self-awareness.

Notably, the term "machine" is used differently today than in Descartes' time, and there is no analog for it at all in the time of these Gnostic writers. However, the notion of control can extend this comparison further. The typical Cartesian notion of "machine" implies a complete understanding of the motion of the machine, while also having it be under complete control, providing some useful benefit to the controller, as with his fanciful daughter-doll. There is a sense of a "nothing but," in that it is lacking autonomy and intelligence, and this can be horrifying. In each of these senses, a likeness can be seen in the demiurge's original creation of the human, and in how he is able to keep people under his control. Descartes appears to be the latest incarnation of this malevolent ruler, in that he supposedly created the entirety of the modern scientific medical model, which attempts to have every function of the human body, and soul, named and explained, and thereby under a kind of control.

Such individual naming of each part and function presents another specific parallel. Recall that in the Gnostic myth there is a separate ruler for each part and function of the human entity, taking up several pages, and each is named. In one sense, this myth reads like a modern medical textbook, only without Latin names such as Gluteus Maximus, but instead Coptic names, such as "Gormakaiochlabar" (Meyer, 2007, pp. 119–124). The overall impression from both is a detailed inventory of merely loose parts, or, in other words, a kind of reductive mechanistic approach to the human being. This is frequently what is implied by the label "Cartesian" by writers such as Capra and Berman. That is, that the human being can be approached by breaking it down into various smaller parts, and assigning a specific name and ruler to each part. This can also be seen in the modern medical approach of specialization, in which each body part and function has a specialized doctor, who masters just one aspect of the human being. This approach is also frequently included under the "Cartesian" rubric.

This comparison can be extended to modern psychology textbooks as well, especially those in cognitive psychology. These can also resemble a detailed inventory of loose parts, only instead of physical parts being individually and rigorously named, there are psychological entities, such as cognitive pathways, sensory inputs, memory storage units, and retrieval mechanisms. Such a large inventory of mental *things* naturally derives from the "Cartesian" conception of mind, that which Baker and Morris (2002) call the Expansion Thesis (p. 15). The Gnostic myth includes all of the above in one long, wholly depressing account.

Finally, as mentioned before, this detailed inventory is presented heavily in terms of pairs of opposites. The writers of this myth seem to be astonished by the fact that the human body can be so easily divided up between right and left. No less than 19 body parts are broken down in this manner, and each of these has at least two rulers. One appears to have merely formed them, while the other "activates them" (Meyer, 2007, pp. 119–123). It is probable that the authors regarded this division in the same way as they did human culture, in which people of the right struggle alongside those of the left, both helpless against the ruler of them all. Thus, a line from another text has a possible double meaning, reflecting both this strife and the polarity of the body. "God, the ruler of the realms and the powers, angrily divided us" (p. 347).

Feminism and ecology

As demonstrated earlier, the fields of feminism and ecological studies seem to have a higher interest than most on residual Cartesian influence. This is of course not coincidental, as the earth has historically been attributed with feminine characteristics. Because of this, regardless of its legitimacy, the burden of voicing environmental concerns has fallen to many feminist theorists, and Descartes is often singled out as a common enemy. Interestingly, this modern sentiment, as a combination, may have a specific antique root.

Perhaps it all starts from the beginning, in which the demiurge's very first experiences are troubles with the feminine. After being borne tragically out of Sophia's passions, his first act is to take "great power" away from her (Meyer, 2007, p. 115). From that moment on, this painful separation results in all sorts of neurotic behavior. Occasionally, she tries to correct his errant ways, but this only results in more irrational boasting (p. 191). Even just hearing her voice results in various groanings, feelings of shame, and becoming "deeply distressed" (p. 209).

However, the demiurge does not keep this behavior to himself, as he and his archons frequently act out in an overtly misogynistic fashion. After learning that Eve had transgressed against them, they became greatly agitated and covetous. They seized and defiled her, and many women after her, foully and abominably (Meyer, 2007, pp. 127, 130, 194–195). "They defiled her in ways natural and obscene" (pp. 214–215). Worse, they act to ensure that her future daughters would be forced to submit to them sexually in the same way, producing legions of ignorant offspring (p. 130).

Out of this legacy of neurotic behavior, various environmental crises seem to develop along with it. The archons are as unecological as they are misogynistic. The rulers "selfishly despoil the earth" (Hoeller, 1989, p. 146). And after their various missteps, they come to regret their creation and decide to just destroy it all with the great flood. In typical Gnostic fashion, the humans are not blamed for the flood as much as they are in Genesis. Rather, the flood is presented more as an illegitimate act of eco-terror. And with this act in particular, the rulers show their disdain for both women and earth. They "lusted after the daughters of men," even as the flood is being planned (p. 673). According to one text, Eve's daughter Norea tried to thwart their evil plans, and in response, they try to defile her as well (Meyer, 2007, p. 195). Perhaps Norea was the first eco-feminist, as she tries to protect both the earth and her body from the ruler's wanton and reckless acts.

Finally, as is fitting for the age of the rulers, the myth predicts that their selfish wars will result in an ecological apocalypse. "The seas will dry up. . . the springs will stop giving water," and "the sun will stop shining" (Meyer, 2007, p. 400). In another text, there will be thunder and mountains catching fire. "The earth will be drunk from the blood that is poured out. The seas will be troubled by war." In this account, however, the role of the feminine takes up an ambivalent role, with Sophia as both victim and instigator. This is because all of creation is associated with "the firmament of the female" (p. 220). As such, she participates in its ultimate destruction. However, it is to be noted that the majority of the texts emphasize the terrible and foolish actions of the rulers during this overall process.

Solipsism and materialism

One of the truly unique features of the Split Worlds myth is how it diverges into further extremes, the further away it moves from academic philosophy. In the conventional treatment, such as is found in Ryle, the two worlds of Cartesian dualism exist in parallel and are linked by two-way causation. However, in fields outside of similarly focused attention, such as general psychology, the two worlds are often stated as being radically and completely separated from one another. When this notion is added, it seems to facilitate the occurrences of the dual themes of Cartesian Solipsism and Materialism.

Cartesian Solipsism, as I have presented it, is a condition that would result from an excessive focus on private thinking, combined with a radical separation from everything else. The Solipsist Descartes doubts his senses, and everything he has learned, and trusts only his present thinking process, his own private realm of *res cogitans*. There is the notion that this is a sort of philosophical terminus, a radically nihilistic dead-end, in which the subject's thoughts are the only reality. I have already demonstrated the basic parallel of this to the Gnostic demiurge, who loudly declares himself to utterly alone in all of creation.

However, upon close inspection of the Gnostic myth, this kind of radical isolation takes on additional meaning. Again, there is a vast system of higher entities and powers that preceded the creation of the demiurge, and in fact, the demiurge's entire existence and personal characteristics derive from these higher patterns. Further, they continue to exert influence on the events that occur in both heaven and earth. However, again, the demiurge is tragically ignorant of all of this. Or rather, it is perhaps *because* of this ongoing influence that creates and maintains the *feeling* of radical isolation. This will require some further exposition.

Essentially, the demiurge suffers from denial. There must be a lingering memory concerning this heritage, his lost mother, and the higher pattern of the divine Father, from which he was created. As one text notes explicitly, there must have been other gods, for otherwise, there would be no need to proclaim his singular nature so boastfully (Meyer, 2007, p. 117). However, the conditions of his birth are tragic, and therefore this memory must cause him some pain. Rather than confronting this pain, he denies it. And so, it appears that a manifestly false thought of isolation nevertheless becomes real, and, more importantly, the pain of this lost memory seems to only bring about further isolation.

This effect can be seen at the moment of his creation. Even as higher powers call out to him to remind him that he is not alone, he reacts, quite ironically, by insisting all the more loudly that he is indeed alone (Meyer, 2007, p. 196). But the doubt remains. In one text, he even exhorts, "if anything existed before me, let it appear" (p. 209), as if trying to quell his doubt by hoping nothing will happen. But something does indeed happen. An image of a higher power appears in a blinding fashion from above, which both amazes him and causes shame. A whole series of events proceed from this intrusion, which brings further shame. At one point, the lesser archons laugh at the demiurge for having lied with his boasts of isolation. Again, rather than admit his mistake, the demiurge hatches a devious plan to deny it even further. This time, he creates humans as slaves to ensure that there is no longer any interference from the higher powers which might "ruin our work" (p. 212).

However, in a divine twist of irony, these acts of denial seem to be the very means by which the higher powers continue to exert their influence. In one account of human creation, the demiurge is tricked by their instruction, such that he believes that he alone can animate Adam with his breath. But as he blows, Sophia is secretly behind the scenes, actually providing her own breath instead of his own. With the breath of the higher spirit, humans gain the potential to become more enlightened than the demiurge (Meyer, 2007, pp. 124–125). This of course prompts a whole new round of neurotic behavior, creating a litany of ills for humans to suffer under (pp. 125–130). All of this is therefore a hypostasized idea of isolation superimposed on top of a continuing influence from beyond, but this tension only leads to the *idea* of isolation growing in strength. Further, this leads to actions from the archons that make the continuing influence from above harder to see.

Given this, it is worth reconsidering the Gnostic's legendary hatred of matter. It is commonly thought that Gnosticism is wholly antagonistic toward matter, and therefore the earth and body. There are certainly grounds to support this, but such a reading neglects a large amount of material concerning Gnostic distaste for heaven, or soul, the favored purview of the demiurge. Matter was certainly not loved by the Gnostics, but it was also not an active threat. The body was indeed considered a prison (Meyer, 2007, p. 125), but would not a prisoner blame the law more than the iron bars? Also, it is noted that demiurge did much harm by creating an especially pernicious "phony spirit."

From this perspective, it is the demiurge's flawed *thinking* that creates the flawed cosmos, and this is what the Gnostics were primarily concerned with liberating themselves from. "Our struggle is not against flesh and blood but against the authorities of the world and the spirits of wickedness" (Meyer, 2007, p. 191). This line is actually written by St. Paul in the canonical New

Testament, and for whatever reason, the Gnostic author agreed with him on this point, copying it word for word. Further, another writer advises, "do not fear the flesh *and* do not love it" [italics added] (p. 172). This is because the flesh is but a mere tool of the demiurge's evil plans. In another text, it is indicated that a human who has transcended the ruler's control may wear the flesh with no further problems, perhaps even wearing it with grace (p. 128).

There are many other instances in the myth in which the primary, problematic activity is thinking, and this error extends throughout heaven and earth. One section makes this clear, with a steady blame list of flawed psychic activity. The ruling powers derive from that singular, flawed, "presumptuous thought." They are very proud of themselves, because they are images of the higher powers, but in reality, they have no substance of their own, being only "phantoms, shadows, and illusions." They belonged only to "this empty thought." And again, because "they thought" of themselves as alone, they become disobedient and rebellious. Further, they become victims of their own desires, lust, and fantasies (Meyer, 2007, p. 74).

Also, the demiurge's thought acts as a kind of meta-substance, that seems to transcend both soul and body, heaven and earth. The two realms share the "thought which lies between them, and gives them a common economy" (Meyer, 2007, p. 88). This economy is made up of the two lower orders, which are under his complete command and control. And as he sees it all, he is happy, because he thinks he accomplished it all, "by his own thoughts" (pp 84–85).

However, simply locating the real blame with thinking does not make the problem go away. The Gnostics understood that thinking becomes its own reality, as real as any material substance. "The thought of these others was not idle. . . the things they think about also become their offspring," and this results in all sorts of unpleasantries, such as "fighters, warriors, troublemakers, [rebels], disobedient folks who love to dominate" (Meyer, 2007, p. 75).

It is from this effect that Cartesian Materialism can be seen. The demiurge's thinking process not only isolates him but, at the same time, creates a general state of confusion and chaos by which the spiritual substance can be further hidden. Because the demiurge is so heavily invested in his own lie, he must keep the secret of higher powers hidden from all. If humans were to ever realize their own relationship with the higher powers, the archons' entire system of reality, a system of thinking, would be undone. "Thus all of creation has been blinded so that none might know the God that is over them all" (Meyer, 2007, p. 130).

To maintain this system of ignorance, the rulers devise a system of control that can be considered an early form of Materialism. They present an unending procession of distractions to keep human attention away from Spirit and focused on "things of the world" (Meyer, 2007, p. 194). Humans were "bound with dimensions, times, and seasons." The rulers took the daughters of men for themselves and filled the bodies of the other women with evil. "They brought gold, silver, gifts, copper, iron, metal, and all sorts of things. . . . In this way all creation was forever enslaved" (p. 130). In one passage, the creator is imagined as a malicious fisherman, and humans are the fish. The "adversary is on the lookout for us and is lying in wait for us," and "is delighted to consume us," much like Dennett's Cartesian Theater. Only the ruler's lure is the "the stuff of this world." Humans are tempted by any material thing, and only one bite brings them into slavery. "He introduces the desire for an article of clothing. . . and then love of money, pride, vanity, envy rivaling envy, beauty of body, and covetousness" (pp. 386–387).

Thus, for the Gnostic, perhaps matter itself is not evil, but material-*ism* is. It is the preferred tool of a flawed creator to keep humans in bodily control, and within bodily desires for other material things. This characterization has much in common with the various conceptions of Cartesian Materialism. Capra, in particular, demonstrates this when he describes modern consumerism, and the pursuit of the ideal body image, as direct descendants of the Cartesian legacy. He also claims that this legacy has "led us" to assume that our senses show us the true nature of things, thereby keeping us in a restricted view of reality. Thus, Capra's choice of words is almost identical to that of the various lures of the malicious fisherman of Gnosticism.

It is also very revealing that Capra presents this critique in terms of the *influence on us from Descartes*, rather than in terms of Descartes himself. Capra seems to be half-aware that this would be problematic because he does also state that Descartes rejected his body and sensory experience, and would therefore be anything but materialistic himself. Still, he is able to critique both Solipsism and Materialism, two very different ideas, but both "Cartesian," by splitting them apart in time. That is, he attributes the former to Descartes, and the latter to Descartes' resultant influence. In other words, it is because Descartes rejected the body and identified with thinking, that we are all now today trapped in Materialism. This has a very strong resemblance to the Gnostic myth, in that the demiurge first identified himself with solipsistic thinking, if in tragic error, and in order to provide cover for this error, had to keep humans in a material prison.

It is in this way that the Gnostic myth demonstrates a remarkable ability to relate two diametrically opposed philosophical principles. Rather than being mutually exclusive, these two modalities are part of a continuous fabric of the demiurge's existence. His "authority of matter" is coincidental to his feelings of solipsistic isolation. His thinking is only of himself, and immediately afterwards, he separates heaven and earth, with both being from the one "matter" (Meyer, 2007, pp. 204–205). Further, his desire to contain the fullness of reality in his own thought leads directly to a restrictive worldview, a kind of frozen reality. His unconscious longing for the higher realms "*hardened* for him and remained in him" [italics added] (p. 74). And such hardening from ignorance is pervasive. "Ignorance of the (higher) Father brought terror and fear, and terror *grew dense* like a fog, so that no one could see" [italics added] (p. 36). Thus, the solipsist thinking process of the demiurge is closely correlated with strongly materialistic themes, as if both are aspects of one and the same process. Naturally, this conception of the problem is only possible in a tripartite cosmos, consisting of spirit, soul, and body. In the Gnostic view, the spiritual substance is lost or hidden in a single mixture, consisting of a chaotic blend of soul and body.

Gnostic transcenders

The Gnostic outlook for humanity is certainly grim, but there is hope. The spiritual substance is well-hidden, but hidden is better than missing. And although the rulers are powerful, the Gnostic exegesis is unambiguous in one respect: There are gods higher and more powerful than them. This was revealed to the demiurge himself when he dared one of them to appear. The task for humans is therefore to seek out such help, such that the hidden spark of the Spirit can be liberated.

Crucially, the form of such help is nothing less than a radical Savior, a radiant being of pure Spirit, more powerful than God himself. A classic Gnostic text ends with a hymn of the Savior, exalting his abilities to descend into the underworld three times, before vanquishing the rulers. From this act of salvation, a human can gain protection from both the "angels of misery" and "the demons of chaos" (Meyer, 2007, p. 131). Another text emphasizes the healing of the original separation. "The separation of male and female was the beginning of death." But the Savior comes "to heal the separation that was from the beginning and reunite the two, in order to give life to those who dies through separation and unite them" (p. 175).

It is also emphasized that help comes from the radical beyond, beyond mere human comprehension. "They came from different realms" (Meyer, 2007, p. 219). When the great revealer comes, he will speak in parables, and in 72 languages (p. 397). Finally, it will not happen soon, but "after three ages," at which time "the true human" will appear, to free humans from their "blind thought" (p. 198). This will be accompanied by various apocalyptic events. In addition to the ecological collapse, noted earlier, Sophia has the power to undo heaven as well. "The heavens of the gods of chaos will collapse upon one another and their powers will be consumed. . . . The chief creator's heaven will fall and split in half" (p. 220). Perhaps it is fitting that the demiurge's original splitting becomes his final undoing, being split itself.

This is clearly a religious prophecy concerning the fulfillment of some radically divine plan. Again, such action comes from a deity higher than even God, higher than all of known reality, far beyond mere body and soul. It is therefore quite understandable why there have been so many Cartesian Transcenders. Such heroes as Wittgenstein, Kant, and Einstein were all hailed in heroic terms, and yet could never quite measure up. The Gnostic myth has an answer for this. It might suggest that we are dealing with a divine prophecy, but crucially, this has not yet been fulfilled. These thinkers were geniuses, but still merely human, and could therefore never fully free us from the Cartesian grip.

Summary

In summary, I have presented here a wide range of mythic stories, which collectively have strong resemblances to the overall myth of the Cartesian Split. In general, there are two types of myths that have been referenced, and these roughly correlate to the two aspects of the Cartesian Split myth: The Mirrored Worlds and the Split Worlds. The first are those in which a new world is created via a separation of substances, with a distinct but permeable threshold, and retaining interaction. This is usually established by a culture-hero, acting against the gods, and discussed in generally positive terms, although negative elements may be presaged. Also, the two worlds are presented as opposites to each other. The second type is the overall Gnostic myth, with some antecedents in Plato. In this type, there is also an original separation in creation, but the negative elements are brought to the forefront. Also, this separation is performed by a god who is not a culture-hero, but who guards over the separation and maintains it, to humanity's detriment. There is still a threshold, but it is a tragic threshold. Also, there is a sense of another, even more primary threshold, guarding the entrance to a third world. The opposites are contained in the first two worlds, but there is a sense that the third world is beyond all opposites. Based upon these mutual lines of continuity, the Split Worlds is suggestive of some kind of a condition that directly follows the Mirrored Worlds.

References

Baker, G. P., & Morris, K. J. (2002). *Descartes' dualism*. London, UK: Routledge.

Bordo, S. (1987). *The flight to objectivity: Essays on Cartesianism and culture*. Albany, NY: State University of New York Press.

Campbell, J. (1973). *The hero with a thousand faces* (2nd ed.). Princeton, NJ: Princeton University Press.

Cottingham, J. (1998). Introduction. In J. Cottingham (Ed.), *Descartes* (pp. 1–27). Oxford, UK: Oxford University Press.

Hardacre, H. (2017). *Shinto: A history*. New York, NY: Oxford University Press.

Hoeller, S. A. (1989). *Jung and the lost gospels: Insights into the Dead Sea scrolls and the Nag Hammadi library*. Wheaton, IL: Theosophical.

Jonas, H. (1972). *The Gnostic religion: The message of the alien god and the beginnings of Christianity* (2nd ed.). Boston, MA: Beacon Press.

Meyer, M. (Ed.). (2007). *The Nag Hammadi scriptures*. San Francisco, CA: HarperSanFrancisco.

Meyer, M., & Pagels, E. H. (2007). Introduction. In M. Meyer (Ed.), *The Nag Hammadi scriptures* (pp. 1–13). San Francisco, CA: HarperSanFrancisco.

Pinch, G. (2004). *Egyptian mythology: A guide to the gods, goddesses, and traditions of ancient Egypt*. Oxford, UK: Oxford University Press.

Plato. (1952a). Symposium. In B. Jowett (Trans.), *Great books of the western world, vol. 7 Plato* (pp. 149–173). Chicago, IL: William Benton, Encyclopedia Britannica.

Plato. (1952b). Timaeus. In B. Jowett (Trans.), *Great books of the western world, vol. 7 Plato* (pp. 442–477). Chicago, IL: William Benton, Encyclopedia Britannica.

Rodis-Lewis, G. (1998). Descartes and the unity of the human being. In J. Cottingham (Ed.), *Descartes* (pp. 197–210). Oxford, UK: Oxford University Press.

Thomas, C. C. S. (1996). *The allure of determinacy: Truth and Cartesian certainty* (Doctoral dissertation). Retrieved from ProQuest Dissertations and Theses. (UMI 9625960)

von Franz, M.-L. (1972). *Patterns of creativity mirrored in creation myths*. Dallas, TX: Spring.

Zeyl, D. (2014). Plato's Timaeus. In E. N. Zalta (Ed.), *The Stanford encyclopedia of philosophy*. Retrieved from: https://plato.stanford.edu/archives/spr2014/entries/plato-timaeus/

Chapter 6

Psychological interpretation

In the first chapters, I explored in depth the notion of a modern myth, currently roaming the halls of Western academia, in the form of a cultural complex, revolving around a highly exaggerated historical figure. This myth is mostly unconscious, in that it is not recognized as a myth or a complex, but believed to be historical fact. I then showed that this figure has much more in common with mythic figures, such as the Gnostic demiurge, than a man named René Descartes. However, thus far I have only briefly introduced the basic psychological dynamics that can make such a mythological distortion possible. This chapter will explore such notions in more detail.

In the case with Ash, these will be the notes recorded privately in the therapist's notebook. It is generally not helpful to discuss psychological details with someone who is struggling with such a compelling story, operating in the depths of the mind. In practice, these deeper levels generally do not respond well to technical terminology.

Nevertheless, the therapist must eventually resort to some kind of psychological theory. If nothing else, it is helpful in order to visualize the problem in abstract terms, perhaps to gain some critical distance. It is also needed to make better sense of the historical parallels. Without a proper psychological understanding, such parallels may seem arbitrary or coincidental, or at best, curious. However, under the cover of archetypal theory, such parallels are essential toward gaining a better understanding of the present dynamics. It is exactly on the basis of archetypes that the musings of a long-dead French philosopher can become the stuff of myth, hundreds of years later, and on new continents, resembling myths from ancient times.

To understand this, Jung argued that the human mind is not a *tabula rasa,* but rather, is born with a full slate set of inherited archetypes. These are *a priori* conditioning factors in the unconscious psyche, that tend to express themselves through mythological, or "primordial," images. Archetypes are defined as being shared by all humans, and throughout all of human history, and so there are always comparisons possible from modern ideas, from any discipline, back to ancient myths. Specifically, Jung (1918/1970) argued that archetypes are not images themselves, but rather inherited *potentials* to form such images. These potentials are inherited anew with every human being, along with our common brain structure (pp. 10–11). They can be understood in this context as latent structures, lying in wait, until the appropriate situation activates them, at which time they spontaneously form psychic images. These images are formed using whatever material is available in the conscious mind, and yet conforming to certain recognizable patterns. It is in this way that the capacity to form demiurge-like images are common to both modern philosophers and ancient Gnostics alike.

The notion of a psychological commonality is reinforced by the similar dynamics of the two stories throughout time. The Gnostics appeared to have taken a Mirrored Worlds creation myth, which was generally positive, and embellished it with a much darker tone. The two worlds no longer peacefully interact but are locked in an unending strife. In one case, there was no possibility of upward movement. The only hope was a transcendence of opposites, brought about by unknown forces.

In modern times, we see the same pattern played out in philosophy. Originally, there was the Legend of Descartes, who once upon a time momentously unleashed the Two Worlds doctrine, subsequently dictating the agenda for all subsequent debate. Although problematic, it was still a good story, worth repeating and thinking about. This story was then exaggerated and twisted to the point where it became a terrible, all-pervasive threat. The Two Worlds now consisted of every kind of opposites, bitterly fighting against each other, until the end of time. Now, there are the extremes of Solipsism and Materialism, with misogynism and ecological destruction to boot. In both cases, then, the Split Worlds is a continuation, or twisted expansion, of the Mirrored Worlds, due to some common psychological dynamic. I will now attempt to name this dynamic, in the same general sequence.

Interpretation of the mirrored worlds

Providing a psychological interpretation of this myth features an inherent difficulty. This is because the source material of this myth was originally presented in already psychological terms, which were themselves the result of existing interpretation. In other words, I am now tasked to interpret an interpretation, while also psychologizing psychology. However, in the midst of all these mundane terms there were clearly mythical ones as well, such as the "Ghost in the Machine," and the notion of common people living tragically in a "bifurcated" reality, the "two worlds." These dramatic statements, combined with all the exaggerations and distortions already presented, indicate that something is in need of further interpretation. Also, Ryle refers to the Cartesian worldview as a myth, only by this, he means it is false. In the Jungian tradition, a myth means that it is symbolic, that something is still unknown. Further, stories of underworlds and spirit worlds have been told and retold by generations of people, all around the world. Such stories give meaning to their lives and help structure their entire conception of reality. Therefore, when these themes show up in a philosophical argument, and are denounced as false, it is certainly worth reconsideration.

In general, the depth psychology tradition understands such stories as being symbolic of the basic structural form of the psyche, the dual realms of the conscious and unconscious mind. Specifically, the day-world is interpreted as the conscious mind, with the underworld, spirit-world, or world of the dead, as referring to the unconscious. Freud's motto for his seminal *The Interpretation of Dreams* is a quote from Virgil's Aeneid: "If I cannot bend the Higher Powers, I will move the Infernal Regions." This is a classic Two Worlds image. It is also consistent with the hero's journey in that consciousness must leave the day-world, and descend to the underworld, in order to solve the problem at its root. This overall sentiment extends also throughout the Jungian tradition in the form of the *Nekyia,* or undersea journey.

However, the specific spatial assignments of these terms are not necessarily fixed. In other words, the unconscious is not always "below," as Freud's superego is an unconscious influence acting from "above." Similarly, Jung was deeply concerned about the unconscious influence of ideologies, or all the various "-isms." These are abstract, mental constructs, rather than bodily instincts, but still act unconsciously. The important thing to note is that the overall schema of the Two Worlds, and especially of the Mirrored Worlds, is uniquely evocative of the nature of consciousness, the day-world, and its relationship to the other-world, the shadowy underworld of the unconscious. In the present study, it was the legendary Descartes who first marked out the newly discovered inner world of consciousness, by planting a flag, inscribed by the words *Cogito Ergo Sum.*

Becoming conscious of consciousness

First, an attempt must be made to clarify the term *consciousness.* This is an extraordinarily difficult term to define, and what follows is my interpretation of Jung's usage of the term. In this sense, it does not refer directly to a state of waking versus sleeping, nor is it in reference to simple sentience, such as response to stimuli, found in all forms of life. Rather, it can be defined in the most general sense as a certain mode of psychic activity which is best demonstrated by a statement such as "I am aware of something." Note that with this definition, I am not equating "consciousness" with "awareness," which is famously noted to be a circular definition. Rather, I am emphasizing the special role of the linguistic statement that best demonstrates it. Therefore, language plays an important role in consciousness, and this necessarily implies something unique to humans, insofar as humans have the most developed linguistic systems. Certainly, animals have languages too, but there are no recorded animal mythologies of the Two Worlds, describing the nature of consciousness. Therefore, my attention is directed to the faculty of human consciousness, which is best expressed in the mythological language of the day-world, over and against the underworld.

Further, consciousness, in this sense, does not necessarily correlate to conventional truth. In other words, the statements "I am aware of that green tree," and "I am aware that I was abducted by aliens," are both equally valid statements of consciousness, even if the latter can be proved to be impossible, from a strictly positivistic point of view. Consciousness, in my usage, is therefore an extremely subtle process that is common between these two seemingly different statements.

Finally, consciousness is difficult to define because every definition is itself an act of consciousness. This would be the case even if consciousness, as a subject, is denied. In other words, the viewpoint of scientific materialism might say that consciousness is nothing but an epiphenomenon of the brain, as if it can be wholly reduced and explainable by way of brain chemicals. It is implied from this that the subjective experience of consciousness, as an original experience, is somewhat of an illusion. And so, someone such as Dennett might state: "I deny the existence of consciousness," and yet this statement itself, in my interpretation, is an act of consciousness. This is because the "I" of this statement, in this case Dennett, would necessarily have to be *conscious* of spurious evidence for (conventional) consciousness. In this sense, it is difficult to define something that you can never fully detach yourself from, to view it objectively. For these reasons, consciousness may be best expressed in symbolic form, such as in myth, rather than a definition. Overall, I wish to emphasize that my usage of the term is different from that which is found in most existing interpretations of Cartesian philosophy, and this is another reason which necessitates a new interpretation.

There are four primary characteristics of consciousness, as I define it. These are the differentiation of opposites, the threshold of consciousness, the interaction across the threshold, and the establishment of certainty. Each of these will now be explored in more detail, along with the corresponding images from the Mirrored Worlds myths.

Differentiation of opposites

For Jung, every act of consciousness is a differentiation between opposites. This can be demonstrated by using a rather mundane example. The positive statement "the tree is green," can only be made when juxtaposed to, and raised above, any other statement that negates it. These might be, for example, statements such as "the tree is not green," "the tree is red," or "the tree is burnt." All such latter statements must be withheld, in order for the positive statement to be established and maintained. Also, all of these statements of negative form may remain undifferentiated from each other, in the unconscious. In other words, I do not have to differentiate between any of the various negative statements, in order to assert the positive statement. The difference between "red" and "burnt" is inconsequential while asserting "green." It can be seen from this example that consciousness and the unconscious are both engaged in every moment of conscious psychic activity, in the same way that positive and negative charges are involved in every instance of the flow of electricity.

It must be understood, however, that consciousness is not the rote opposite of unconsciousness. Rather, these two realms are the structures by which any possible pair of opposites can be constituted in the conscious mind. It is only in this respect that, for Jung (1928/1969), the unconscious invariably "behaves in a compensatory or complementary manner toward the conscious" (pp 69–71).

This act of differentiation is why there are so many pairs of opposites in all of the general Two Worlds myths that I have referenced. In particular, Empedocles' notion of Neikos is exemplary, in that the original separation of primal elements, precedes the creation of everything else, that is, any other pair of opposites. This is also commonly symbolized, in the other myths, by the metaphors of first substances, such as heaven and earth, or the first world parents. It is therefore easy to see how any possible pair of opposites, and therefore all forms of conscious psychic activity, can be derived from such an original separation, and this is also expressed in the myths themselves. The most frequent of these pairs are day from night, life from death, heaven from earth, mother from father, and male from female. In the more modern form of the Cartesian Split, it shows up in Ryle, in which the two worlds take the form of four primary pairs of opposites: Inner and outer, immaterial and material, certain and uncertain, and private and public. From this, the idea of a fundamental Split has expanded greatly in scope, as shown in all the other pairs of opposites, presented in the other sources.

Crossing the threshold

As demonstrated earlier, a positive statement of consciousness must be clearly demarcated against all the various negative statements. If "the tree is green" is too close to the "the tree is red," or any of the other negative statements, then the positive image cannot be held to be true. A threshold must be maintained. From another frame of reference, hypnosis is commonly understood to weaken the threshold of consciousness. Under such a state, the subject is unusually receptive to unconscious contents, or may not be able to formulate a string of coherent statements. The situation may also be similar to that of a sleepwalker, with a similarly compromised threshold. In these cases, positive and negative statements can be imagined to be too close together. In order for consciousness to proceed, a threshold must be maintained to elevate and isolate conscious contents from all the others.

For Freud, such a threshold is manifested continuously by all of the various repressions and defense mechanisms, protecting us from the underworld, or the "seething cauldron" of instincts. The threshold is also guarded over by the mysterious dream censor, and also shows up as the incest taboo. Such guardians act to prevent the instinctual pleasure-seeking urges of the Id from breaking out into the open, into the realm of ego-consciousness and the reality principle.

Jung inherited this overall structure, although he preferred to express the threshold in a more abstract form, consisting of quantities of psychic energy, and not just sexual libido. It is from this schema that I drew my example. In this schema, all contents of consciousness must have a sufficient amount of psychic energy, in order to rise above the threshold of consciousness, suppressing the lower energy value of all the various negative statements. For both Freud and Jung, however, the threshold was seen as an absolute necessity, for the complete absence of it would likely constitute a severe psychosis.

Such a defined threshold can be found in the previously referenced myths, one that demarcates the two realms from each other. This is expressed by such images as the entrance to Plato's cave, or a special geographic feature leading to the underworld, such as the river Lethe, or Izanagi's boulder. In all cases, the threshold has a certain firmness, even though there are certain instances of passage across it. However, such a passage is always accompanied by some kind of a special ritual, or some other unusual event, such as Persephone's abduction to the underworld. In the case of Ryle, crossing the threshold between the outer world to the inner world requires a complete shift of the mode of perception; from fuzzy perception through the senses, in public, to clear perception using introspection, in private.

Mutual causation

Depth psychology understands the two worlds as being linked by two-way causation across the threshold. For Freud, this is best seen by the various neuroses, most famously the Freudian "slip of the tongue." These and other neuroses are therefore active agents from the unconscious, crossing the threshold to cause certain events in consciousness. Correspondingly, these neuroses are themselves caused by an original conscious repression of the Id. Further, only analysis, including work that must be done by the ego, can eliminate this unresolved tension, thereby causing the desired change in the unconscious.

Jung agreed with Freud on this overall mode of causation but added some additional modalities. For Jung, complexes also serve an adaptive role, which features further two-way causation. Complexes can serve to correct and modify a consciousness that has become unbalanced, and out of adaptation to reality. In this model, consciousness causes a psychic imbalance from an excessive reliance on its own contents, or in Jung's terminology, excessive "one-sidedness." Complexes then rise up from the unconscious in order to cause a correction in the original conscious course. This naturally depends on a constant flow of information and causality between the two realms.

Overall, such causation can also be seen reflected in the classic Two Worlds myths. Generally, spirits cause hauntings in the day-world, and shamans can cause spirits to stop. Plato's souls both cross Lethe and yet remember, and similarly, souls cross Izanagi's boulder both ways. It is noted that most critics agree that Descartes insisted on mutual causation, even as they mock such "Cartesian Interactionism." Again, this would be in the same way as they might deride such fairy tales and myths.

The one world of certainty

In all of the Two Worlds myths, one world is generally considered to be more certain and stable than the other world, and this generally represents consciousness. In this case, the interpretation is self-evident. The day-world is the world of light, and light is the universal symbol of consciousness.

In most of the myths I have referenced, the day-world of consciousness is the same world as that which is perceived through the physical senses. However, this is not universally the case. Consciousness in its purest form is not inherently tied to sensible reality, as defined earlier. "I am aware of being abducted by aliens" is a valid statement of consciousness, even though it may not have a verifiable empirical basis.

Therefore, we might expect versions of the Two Worlds myth in which the sensible world is uncertain, and therefore not the same as the light-world. This is indeed the case, such as with the Buddhist doctrine of *Maya*. From this view, the world of physical things, or forms, is recognized as the world of illusion, being surreal and uncertain. Usually, this insight is said to be achieved by a solitary enlightened figure who has withdrawn from conventional reality and the senses, such as a meditating yogi, or guru. Such a figure is easily imagined to be in some remote place, like on the top of a mountain, or in other words, above the mundane world. From this vantage point, the real world, a new world, is found only in the midst of conscious contemplation of the mind itself.

Interestingly, this specific image of the guru is actually closer to the case of the Mirrored Worlds myth than any other I have referenced so far. It is, after all, the Legendary Descartes who was imagined to be sitting alone in a stove-heated room, withdrawn from the senses, when he received the grand inspiration, and subsequently wrote down the *Meditations*. The inner world that was created by this Legendary work, the infamous *res cogitans*, is immaterial, private, and yet apprehended with absolute certainty. Correspondingly, the outer world is physical, public, and yet the senses conveying these objects are doubtful.

In consideration of this, the psychological interpretation of the Mirrored Worlds myth may carry with it a striking implication, at least for some. When the terms "inner world" and "outer world" are invoked in the Jungian tradition, it is common for consciousness to be associated with "outer," and the unconscious with "inner" (Jacobi, 1968, p. 7,130; Jung & Jaffé, 1989, pp. 4–5). However, in the myth of Cartesian Dualism, it is the opposite. In this case, *consciousness is being represented in this myth by the inner world*. By extension, this also implies that consciousness, in this presentation, is characterized by immateriality, which is different from the usual Jungian usage.

And so, the unique structure of this Mirrored Worlds myth, on close inspection, appears to be somewhat alien, perhaps more of an Eastern nature than many of the myths more familiar to the West, such as Campbell's monomyth. However, I believe this interpretation follows the source material of the present myth most closely.

The creation of consciousness

Whenever a Two Worlds myth is presented in the specific form of a creation myth, it is symbolic not of the creation of any literal world, but of the creation of consciousness itself. In most of the traditional myths, the separation between the two worlds occurs before any kind of recognizable human activity, which symbolizes the notion that the threshold is fundamental. As such, the separation is often effected by some kind of a divine figure, which symbolizes that this structure was developed outside of conscious control. In modern scientific terms, this is likely the result of inhuman evolutionary forces. In other words, no proto-human ever decided to enable conscious activity by first establishing a threshold. It is something that evidently just happened, and we unconsciously inherit it. In the language of myth, such a process is always symbolized by a god.

Put into other terms, a creation myth concerning the separation of the opposites is symbolic of the original emancipation of a differentiated consciousness from a prior state of nondifferentiation, thereby enabling all other basic cognitive functions. Prior to this act of differentiation, all such statements exist, in potential form, in the unconscious, but nothing happens. Hence, any positive statement of consciousness necessarily creates two worlds out of one. The creation myths of this form serve to illustrate the full context of how this condition originates, and how such a condition must be treated. With this overall interpretation, I am following closely existing interpretation by several first-generation Jungians (Edinger, 1984, p. 37; von Franz, 1972, p. 155).

Depth psychology emphasizes that such a separation of worlds is a positive event. Both Freud and Jung believed it to be indispensable for civilization, even if this was necessarily accompanied by the various neuroses of their respective fields. As such, von Franz (1972) explicitly notes the positive tone of most myths of separation (p. 155). This is in spite of the occasionally traumatic overtones, such as those found in the Maori myth. This is to be understood in the sense that, naturally, consciousness must be established, even if it causes some kind of overall psychic disturbance.

Further, it is important to note that the creation of consciousness is an ongoing task. Every new statement of awareness or realization comes in some form of discrimination of opposites, and therefore a separation between a positive statement against its negation (von Franz, 1972, p. 155). As such, creation myths can equally be understood to be symbolic of the ongoing task of creativity, and naturally, in this respect, it is always regarded as a positive act. One can readily see this tendency today, in modern culture, particularly in the various creation myths of Silicon Valley. People seem to love to tell stories about how companies, such as Google, Amazon, and Disney, were formed by a few people in small garages in suburban California (Erlanger & Govela, 2018).

Death at the threshold

However, a truly mythic perspective must not regard all creation as all positive. The creation of consciousness is essential for life, but in order for new life to be created, something must also die. As noted, this was indicated in most of the traditional creation myths. There was always a certain struggle involved in the separation of opposites, which thereby enables consciousness. The pre-existing state of totality must be broken, divided, or even destroyed, and this can be difficult and traumatic. The only difference among the myths is to what degree this struggle is noted. Also, the discarded opposite is sometimes seen to be tragically relegated to the other world, the underworld, and potentially lost, such as the case with Izanami. This creates a sort of necessary tension of psychic existence, and this opposition must eventually be accounted for, even if the more positive creation myths do not seem to directly address it. Overall, this tension symbolizes that consciousness has a double aspect; it is not all positive.

The unmistakable presence of death in creation myths is perhaps the simplest expression that the creation of consciousness is not all positive. This is readily seen in the fact that in most Two Worlds myths, the other world is populated by the dead, and the dead frequently make their presence known in various dark and foreboding ways. However, there is sometimes an additional notion. Perhaps it is exactly death itself, in all of its stark and unfortunate reality, which somehow acts as a stimulant for the creation of consciousness. In other words, consciousness may be life, but death creates consciousness.

This can be seen in the Japanese myth, in that Izanami and Izanagi only settle on their mutual separation by agreeing upon an ongoing exchange of human souls, with the first event being death. It is only after this moment that human culture properly started. Similarly, it is only after Marduk completes his bloody killing of Tiamet that human civilization can start. Overall, the presence of death in this manner is symbolic of humans leaving behind a preconscious state of purely instinctual life, such as that lived by lower animals. Clearly, for animals, death certainly happens, but it is doubtful that they are fully aware of it, or spend much time brooding about it. It is the painful knowledge of death that separates us from animals as conscious human beings, and this notion is powerfully symbolized by the splitting apart of two worlds. Also, this cannot be undone. As Joseph Campbell (1983) writes, in agreement with Spengler and Tolstoy, it was "this awakening to the knowledge of death [that] set man apart from the beasts and the plants... At that instant the consciousness of man fell in two, separated in the awakened mind from the innocence" (p. 25).

Not only can awareness of death be seen as creative of consciousness, but it can also be seen as necessary for ongoing psychic health. An example of this can be found in the ritual of the Day of the Dead, which seems to serve a cultural need. This of course requires a myth of two worlds, one of the dead and one of the living. Although certain aspects of such rituals may be somewhat unsettling to some, it is precisely the awareness of this other reality that provides comfort to the living. Further, this awareness must be ritually re-enacted, as a constant reminder. This is the redeeming notion of the awareness of death, sometimes referred to as the *memento mori*. Overall, it seems that a full awareness of the reality of two worlds, and with it the reality of death, reflects a certain necessary ambivalence regarding the creation of consciousness.

Such an ambivalence can also be readily seen in the myth of Cartesian Dualism, specifically the Mirrored Worlds of philosophy. As noted earlier, every philosophy student is required to be well versed in Cartesian Dualism, even though the vast majority of professors will teach it in a manner in which all the unseemly aspects of it are exposed. All the supposed logical fallacies, contradictions, and dead-ends are demonstrated in plain relief, and this may even serve a therapeutic function to the academic community (Baker & Morris, 2002, p. 3). This therefore could be a modern parallel to the ritual of *memento mori*. Similarly, Bordo emphasizes the need for a close study of Descartes, but only to the extent that this can enlighten us to the painful reality of our separation from the "organic" Middle Ages.

In summary, I consider it highly likely that the Mirrored Worlds is a new creation myth, but unrecognized as such. This is based on the simultaneous lack of consistency with historical facts and the presence of consistency with similar creation myths. This myth has been spontaneously produced from unknown psychic depths but is being expressed in contemporary terms. In this myth, a figure of mythological proportions, commonly referred to as Descartes, has created a new world, the inner world, at the beginning of our modern age. This new world is haunted by the Legendary Cartesian "I," a disembodied something of the substance *res cogitans*, and this has occupied some of our greatest minds ever since, despite all of their misgivings.

Translated into psychological terms, this creation myth signifies that something new has been created, from factors outside of our control, concerning the most basic element of psychic existence. Or rather, something new is being created now. In either case, *some new insight is now available concerning the nature of consciousness, its origins, and perhaps its needs.* Also, the myth states that consciousness, in this case, is characterized by immateriality. Finally, and importantly, the ambivalence of the subject suggests that all is not ideal in the new world of consciousness. Naturally, Descartes the human did not and could not have been involved in the construction of such a myth, but this only serves to reinforce the notion that we are dealing with a myth proper.

Interpretation of the split worlds

The Split Worlds myth has many unique features, which require additional interpretation. These features are likely a result from being formed in a community of scholars outside of dedicated philosophy. As such, it was generated from sources at least one degree further removed from Descartes' actual writings, and this may have allowed for more freedom of expression. With this free play of fantasy, new themes were able to be added to the Mirrored Worlds myth. Central to this is the new sense of a radical split, with no interaction between the two worlds. Also, there are the themes of Ecological Crisis, Subjective Difficulties, Reduction and Isolation, and the conflicting themes of Solipsism and Materialism. Finally, there is not much ambivalence left, the entire notion is outright rejected, without even meriting a glance at the primary sources. Although all of these themes have direct antecedents in the Mirrored Worlds myth, they are often expressed more strongly, and in more dramatic terms, in the Split Worlds myth.

In spite of these novelties, the overall continuity strongly suggests that the Split Worlds myth concerns the same subject. This is further reinforced in the continuity between all the myths I have used for amplification. That is, the Gnostic myth clearly incorporates within it all the core elements of the more traditional Two Worlds myths. It is exactly as if the Gnostic myth was formed in the same fashion as the Split Worlds myth. In both cases, a new audience has taken traditional writings and embellished them with several new themes, mostly of a highly dramatic nature, while at the same time casting the entire idea in a much more negative light.

However, these changes certainly do not change the fact that the Split Worlds is still very much a creation myth. If anything, the Split Worlds myth is more of a creation myth than any sources that I have referenced for the Mirrored Worlds. Most academic philosophers recognize some novelty in Descartes' works but generally do not ascribe to it over-arching critical importance. Some see Descartes as not original at all, merely recapitulating ancient skepticism, or elements of Augustine. By contrast, the Split Worlds myth often frames the *cogito* as *the* moment of philosophical history. It is as if everything that happened beforehand was a continuous, uninterrupted process, but this is now separated from us by this momentous Split. A similar feeling is found in the Gnostic myth, which feature much more detailed creation myths, and more versions of them, than found in Genesis.

Of all the novelties of the Split Worlds, it is perhaps this general feeling that stands out, this radical focus on ultimate origins. This will be the first area of focus for interpretation. The overall attitude in both the Split Worlds and Gnostic myths can be summarized succinctly: *Something has gone wrong.* There is some fundamental, tragic flaw in all of known creation. Special attention must therefore be paid to creation myths because the dominant myth of the times is not big enough to explain this fundamental flaw. In other words, the problem of the present world is not some trivial mistake, something easily correctable. No, it must go all the way back to the very creator of the world. For the Gnostics, this was God, for us, Descartes.

I have already demonstrated that Two World creation myths most commonly concern the creation of consciousness. If this new attitude is superimposed upon this, a provisional interpretation of the Split Worlds may now be made. Briefly, the Split Worlds myth suggests that *something has gone very wrong with the creation of consciousness.* In other words, that most basic datum of the human psyche, without which nothing can be said to exist, has somehow lost its most basic integrity.

With such dramatic overtones, making any further interpretations in psychological language is particularly challenging. Interpretations should always tentative, but even more caution should be given in this situation, because of the tentative nature of my source material. The Split Worlds myth, if it even exists as such, may have only been documented for the first time in the present study. It is for this reason that I very carefully laid out the comparisons to a prior mythical structure, to establish a more secure foundation. Although there are certainly still some complexities and mysteries in the Gnostic myth, it at least has the benefit of being already published, along with several decades of critical work by multiple sources. For this reason, it may be helpful to follow the lead of the myth itself, going back to the very beginnings, by working first with the parallels from ancient times.

Gnostic consciousness

Upon reflection, the Gnostic myth is truly innovative in scope. The authors appear to have taken existing Two Worlds mythologies and turned these entire systems around, with three primary movements. First, they made no special distinction between the two inherited worlds. The realm of ideal forms, the upper spheres of astrology, and the heaven of Judaism, were no longer characterized as being sacred, or in any way mysterious. Rather, heaven was just as mundane as earth, populated by animal-gods with all-too-human tendencies. The chief archon was a common fool, no better than poorly skilled craftsman, bungling every attempt at creation. When it came to the people who inherited this structure, the Gnostics saw the heavenly-minded Rights on one side, and earthly-minded Lefts on the other, and were not especially impressed with either.

The second movement was to marginalize the entire conception of reality by adding a third world, the highest and most fundamental world of Spirit. Indeed, this is related to the first movement, as there would be no better way to de-emphasize the role of heaven than to say it is merely an upper-level earth, and not that important in the grand scheme. Further, this new third world was completely unknown, outside of a few Gnostic specialists. This is what made Gnosticism truly radical, befitting of course to a "radical" Cartesian Dualism.

Finally, they showed their disdain for both of the two worlds by ascribing to them endless pairs of unfortunate opposites. Heaven and earth, soul and body, Cain and Abel, light elements and dense elements, left and right, the two lower orders, masculine and feminine, emotions and matter, immaterial and material, are all part of the existing systems of thought, and neither side is shown to be especially interesting. It is as if the authors of the texts want to show how horribly mundane both sides of all known reality really is. Similarly, they give no less than five names to the highest known god, as if to say he is also known in every way possible. For the ancients, to have a name for something carries a special meaning. It is to demonstrate a full knowledge of it or to perhaps even demonstrate mastery over it.

The Gnostic texts appear to want to demonstrate *ad infinitum* that nothing of existing knowledge is ultimately worth anything. The first line of *On the Origin of the World* makes this kind of attitude explicit: "Since everyone, both the gods of the world and people, says that nothing existed before chaos, I shall prove they are all wrong, because they do not know the [origin] of chaos or its root" (Meyer, 2007, p. 203). Recall that "root" is etymologically related to "radical." Radical, indeed.

Once this perspective is gained, it can now be brought back to the psychological notion of consciousness. Recall that with the conventional Two Worlds myths, one of the worlds was indeterminate and mysterious, generally representing the unconscious. However, with the endless descriptive lists of both worlds, one cannot help to suspect that for the Gnostics, *both worlds of creation represent consciousness*. Whereas most Two Worlds myths inspired wonder and awe at the mystery of creation, a Gnostic seems to regard these stories as no more interesting than a two-story house. A Hermeticist might say "as above, so below," with a certain reverence, but a Gnostic might say, "So what? The stuff above is the same awful stuff as that of below."

However, they clearly felt the need to retain the distinction between the two worlds. They could have discarded it entirely, and focused only on the distinction between the worlds of the demiurge and the world of Spirit, but they did not. It is as if they knew that these stories of original separation into two still carried some meaning. Perhaps they only wanted to subvert that meaning, rather than abolish it altogether. In any case, this is fortunate, as it may indicate that the myth reflects some kind of transformation of consciousness over time.

This interpretation holds merit upon regarding the notion of the unconscious. If the Gnostics had such a term, they would have undoubtedly reserved it for the world of Spirit, or the *Pleroma*, which is beyond both heaven and earth. This world was deeply mysterious, unknown to the vast majority, and therefore literally "unconscious." And yet, it was still omnipresent and routinely active, even through the actions of the archons, although, of course, even they were unaware of such activity. Or, perhaps they were unconsciously aware of it, and from this comes all the denials and neurotic activity. Whatever symbolic form the unconscious may take in any myth, it must be surrounded by doubt and mystery. This is certainly not the case with the demiurge and heaven. This realm and all the archons' nefarious deeds are explicated in astonishing detail. Fittingly, it is to be noted that the term *Pleroma* is interpreted as the unconscious in the Jungian tradition today (Hoeller, 1982, pp. 69–70). This point is almost made explicit by Jung himself in his Gnostic-inspired *Seven Sermons to the Dead* (Jung & Jaffé, 1989, p. 379).

In summary so far, we might well be able to imagine how a psychologically minded Gnostic might interpret their own complicated mythology. It might proceed something like the following: Listen to all these stories about the original separation of light from darkness, heaven from earth, the above from below. This must be important; probably related to our ability to know anything. But people have been telling these stories for centuries and the world is still a mess. Whoever performed this original separation did not know what they were doing, and now here we are, with the two lower orders locked in eternal strife. There must be something else that we are unaware of. A Savior will come.

Such a crude paraphrase may seem highly spurious, but may yet be useful. It may shed some light on a strikingly similar story in the modern era. We might imagine today a harsh critic of Descartes, a proponent of the Split Worlds myth, pondering something quite similar. One might say: Look at all these philosophy experts go on and on about how Descartes created two worlds, creating the whole new inner world, displacing the Middle Ages. It must be important, probably foundational to the whole modern notion of consciousness. But the experts have debated both sides of this divide for centuries, and the world is still a mess. Descartes must not have known what he was doing, and now all the opposites are forever split apart. There must be something else. Some academic somewhere must be a Heroic Transcender.

Atomic consciousness

The similarity of these two stories, however haphazard, nevertheless invites an extension of the Gnostic interpretation. That is, if the Gnostic worlds both represent consciousness, it is worthwhile to see if this notion can be profitably applied to its modern incarnation, the Split Worlds of Descartes.

As documented earlier, the Cartesian Split is not just between body and mind, but between every conceivable pair of opposites. An initial impression of such long lists might be that it is merely a curious oddity. However, working with this new interpretation may bring insight to this phenomenon. It is to be recalled that both sides of every pair of opposites represented a manifestly known, or *conscious*, quality, much as it seems in the Gnostic myth. Perhaps the best example of this was the Spuybroek (1999) article, which featured the Split between Europe-America, Floor-Wall, Program-Form, Action-Perception, Plan-Elevation, and Feet-Eyes (p. 13). Although some of my sources did mention pairs of opposites such as conscious versus unconscious, and similarly matter versus spirit, I believe it is seen in the original context that even these latter qualities represent some kind of current field of knowledge. For example, the Freudian unconscious is now very well known in the academy, as well as the phenomenology of spirit.

The overall impression one should glean from these long lists is that they are symmetrical. The Spuybroek list would have exactly the same effect if the order within each of the pairs were reversed, and this is the case with virtually all such pairs. I believe the meaning of this is that the *Split represents the over-specialization of knowledge*, or too many instances of consciousness. In other words, we have too many experts too narrowly focused on one topic each, with minimal opportunities for collaboration. Perhaps the exemplary Cartesian Split in this respect is Maguire's (1997) "rupture between science and wisdom" (p. 69). I consider both these pursuits to be conscious activities, but there is of course precious little interaction between academic scientists and spiritual mystics. From a certain perspective, all these divisions reflect individual activities of consciousness that are isolated from each other.

Once this is seen, this suggestion flows easily to other primary themes, first noted in the abstracts. One of these was Reduction and Isolation, which was nominally observed to be the viewpoint of materialistic physics, in which the entire universe is nothing but individually atoms bouncing around each other. But from a psychological perspective, each of these atoms could be taken to represent an individual activity of consciousness. In the mechanistic paradigm, any activity can be broken down into the smallest parts in order to understand it. Similarly, in the academy, every field of knowledge is understood best by isolated areas of subject matter experts. However, any kind of systemic insight, one that might be revealed through creative collaboration, may be missing. This is likely also related to the theme of Limitations of Expression.

Another theme to be revisited is that of the Dominant Paradigm. Earlier, I pointed out the incredulity of the notion that a failed 17th-century philosophy could become the dominant view of the entire world today. However, if such a worldview is reimagined as the sum-total of individual activities of consciousness, it makes more sense. Every single specialist in any field is obviously exercising knowledge, that is, consciousness. Thus, it was very meaningful and fitting that Kelso (2015) defined the Cartesian Split as "that fateful division that now dominates all branches of *knowledge*" [italics added] (para. 2).

Finally, the theme of Over-rationality takes on new meaning, as this is just another way to say over-consciousness. What pulled that theme together was that they were all examples of simply thinking too much, or in other terms, *knowing* too much. That is, the only problem may be becoming too much of an expert in your own field, without taking a step back, to evaluate the bigger picture. It is becoming increasingly clear to many in the academy that this is an unhealthy and unproductive practice. This sentiment may be the link to yet another theme, that of Subjective Difficulties. Remarkably, it is from this theme that we saw Pether's (1999) "Cartesian split subject," which is another way to imagine two halves of consciousness, and also Berman's (1981) near equivalence of "Cartesian" with schizophrenia. This latter term, it is to be noted, means literally "split-mind."

Inside the split

In summary so far, it does appear as if the Split Worlds myth is similar to the Gnostic myth in that both worlds are reflective of consciousness, and neither is especially related to the unconscious. Also, the impression from both is that excessive specialization has become problematic and limiting. However, there is one aspect of the Split Worlds myth that stands out and poses a particular problem for this provisional interpretation. This is the overwhelming emphasis on the *radical* split between the opposites. That is, the two worlds no longer exist side by side, they are not related in form, and they *do not interact* with each other. Rather, they are precluded from mutual interaction on account of their radical separation, the fundamental difference between these two fundamentally different substances.

This notion is not readily found in the Gnostic myth. The two lower orders that constitute the known world are always interacting with each other. Cain and Abel are always fighting, the archons cause trouble on earth, and the human body itself is an animated composite of the right and the left. The demiurge even uses interaction between the worlds to his advantage. Those of heaven are doomed to materialism, and the material ones are doomed to be ruled by heaven, and each side copies each other.

There was, however, one instance in which interaction was prohibited. This was the barrier that kept those on the left, those of matter, from moving up in the hierarchy. Specifically, it was the power that "does not allow them to spread upward to those (on the right, the psychical)" (Meyer, 2007, p. 83). The Gnostics here may have been the first social critics, lamenting the lack of upward mobility. Of course, the higher ones would not want to be demoted, so no barrier is needed to prevent downward mobility.

If this original situation is extended to modern times, as I have already suggested, then the fundamental split between right and left, the notion of non-interaction, does not *really* mean there is no interaction. It may mean that all such interaction is ultimately fruitless. Similarly, today, politicians of the right may endlessly debate politicians from the left, but the situation never *really* improves, at least for many. The right stays right, and the left stays left. Laws are passed, but because there are no meaningful results, it is just as well to say they do not interact. In other words, *there is no* real *causal interaction because nothing ever changes*. The two worlds are forever Split apart, *in spite of* their ongoing interaction.

This interpretation would accord well with the map of themes, originally found in the abstracts. Recall that mind and body were claimed to be radically separated, yet demonstrated in practice to be highly interlinked. Clearly there is enough collaboration in the academy for one field to reference another, with the themes ranging from religious studies to artificial intelligence, if at least to agree on the influence of the Split. And yet, at the same time, there is clearly not enough collaboration, as the Split rages on.

Further, such a dynamic might be the only way to understand the mutual presence of Cartesian Solipsism and Materialism. From a purely philosophical frame of reference, it is difficult if not impossible to understand how these two developments came from a single theorist. However, from a mythical view, a Gnostic view, it may become more apparent. Perhaps half of our scholars are more focused on the immaterial soul, following the example of those on the Right, with the other half focusing on the material body, following the Left. Each of these groups are highly conscious, with perfectly well-thought-out arguments for both sides. Sadly, though, it does not appear they will ever come together. Capra will not agree with Dennett, even though they share a common enemy.

And yet, the Split Worlds myth makes it clear that it is imperative for the two sides to come together. The overall sentiment is that the Split must be transcended, or further, must be outright abolished. This is readily seen in the Heroic Transcender theme, in which their efforts are described in terms such as "destroy" or "explode." There is also an element of finality. Wittgenstein was supposed to sink the ship "once for all," just as Jung's breakthrough was to "put an end" to dualism. The myth is unequivocal: The Split must be overcome, and there is a moment in time in which it can be accomplished. The same pattern occurs in the Gnostic myth, with the coming of the Savior. The fact that this moment has not yet arrived in mundane time does not negate its necessary reality in eternity.

This sentiment shows that the Split Worlds myth is not a conventional Two Worlds creation myth, although it does seem to follow it. Those prior myths are all positive, as the creation of consciousness is indispensable, and the two worlds must be maintained. If those moments of original separation were to be exploded or destroyed, consciousness would be forever lost. What the Split Worlds myth appears to be saying is that consciousness must be created anew, not from reintegration *into* the unconscious, but from a reintegration *of* its own internal contents. This can happen with the threshold between consciousness and the unconscious remaining intact.

In summary, the radical Split between Two Worlds concerns the world of known reality only. In the Gnostic myth, this would be the two worlds that were created and controlled by the demiurge, both heaven and earth. However, as noted, this act of creation was fundamentally flawed. This flaw pervades every aspect of subsequent creation, manifested in every kind of pair of opposites. For the Gnostics, both sides of all of these pairs of opposites were very well known, that is, conscious. Because of this, both sides are sure of their own rightness, but are forever engaged in conflict, until the end of time, because both are bereft of the third world, that of Spirit. Further, their arguments with each other were all part of the demiurge's wicked plans because it was useful for him to stay in power. As such, the two sides of known reality cannot really affect each other, in the sense of being able to ultimately improve the overall situation. Only the coming of the Spiritual Savior, coming from beyond Heaven, can bring salvation. In synthesis of all this, and brought back into psychological language, *the radical Cartesian Split between Two Worlds is a radical split within consciousness itself.*

If this assessment is accurate, it is now necessary to put it into the context of theories of consciousness in the depth psychology tradition. In other words, how does this notion of split consciousness appear in the works of Freud and Jung? Is it novel, or something that has already been developed? As I will show, it appears to something of both.

The splitting of the ego

Notions of splitting run rampant through the whole history of depth psychology. Indeed, there may be no more favorite subject to talk about than things split-off from each other, disassociated, disconnected, separated, or broken down. The task of therapy is, of course, to heal, amend, repair, re-integrate, become whole again. For Jung, the ultimate goal of therapy is to bring the ego into relationship with the central, deepest archetype, the Self. The overall theme of splitting is therefore usually portrayed as a split between consciousness and the deeper levels of the psyche. However, now I am arguing that this particular Split is not that. The splitting of consciousness, as a distinct form of splitting, can be found in the primary literature; however, it requires a bit of filtering and further interpretation.

In the case of Freud, this task has generally already been done, as described in Brook's (1992) "Freud and Splitting." In this article, Brook distinguishes between three different kinds of splitting in Freud's overall body of writings. These are: The splitting of psychic groupings, splitting of representations, and splitting of the ego. Brook suggests that the last form was perhaps the most enigmatic for Freud. Although he approached the subject as early as 1909, it was not properly formulated until 1937. By the end of his life, he may have regarded it as having foundational importance (para. 1). The first two types of splitting cover traditional concepts that have been widely covered in the field (paras. 3, 4). By contrast, the splitting of the ego is somewhat novel. Brook believes it is perhaps even "radically new," something that has not yet been properly understood or appreciated (para. 40–41).

The splitting of groupings may be best understood in terms of classical psychoanalytic repression. It features a collection of psychic entities, which, due to some form of trauma, goes on living a separate existence, interfering with primary consciousness in various ways. Such a grouping is characterized by traits commonly regarded as unconscious, such as lack of sophistication, and rawness of affect. In can be visualized as "horizontal splitting" (Brook, 1992, para. 56), in which the "beneath" lacks conscious qualities. In other words, it is related to the separation between consciousness and the unconscious, which, again, is not what I am considering here.

The splitting of representations may best be understood in terms of object-relations theory, and this form is highly prevalent today (Brook, 1992, para. 4). In this case, a single representation of an object has become split into two, such as Klein's good and bad breast. In this case, there is a sense of a single ego, unaffected by the splitting, which can consciously reflect on both halves of the representation. Therefore, this kind of splitting is also not related to my theme, because the split is all in the "outer" world, having little to do with the subject itself.

The splitting of the ego, however, is very closely related to my suggested theme. It is something that cannot be easily visualized or even conceptualized. In the only dedicated paper on the topic, late in his career, Freud (1938/1964) himself appears to be not even sure what he was dealing with, whether it was old and familiar, or new and puzzling (p. 275). Freud begins his description of this condition in familiar territory, of it being a result of some intolerable conflict between the demand of instincts and the prohibition of reality. However, rather than indulging one and repressing the other, the subject "replies to the conflict with two contrary reactions, both of which are valid and effective" (p. 275). In this example, it can be seen that both sides, although opposite, are equally "conscious," that is, equivalent in believability. Also, Freud's words strongly evoke the idea of an internal split. "On one hand... (the subject) rejects reality... on the other hand, *in the same breath* he recognizes the danger of reality" [italics added] (p. 275). Thus, in this example, there is a simultaneous acknowledgment and disavowal of the same reality. Brook refers to this as "vertical splitting." In other words, a single subject, portrayed with two hands, is divided against himself, in contrast to a still-singular external reality. This formulation of hand versus hand will end up being a useful metaphor, as opposed to head versus body, which would be more indicative of horizontal splitting. There is also the theme of unusual persistence. Freud (1938/1964) states that this is an "ingenious" solution to the conflict, but the solution is short-lived, paid for with a "*rift in the ego which never heals* but which increases as time goes on" [italics added] (p. 276).

Regarding the enigmatic quality of vertical splitting, Freud (1938/1964) states that the splitting of the ego only seems strange to us because we assume that the ego is singular, but in this assumption, we are mistaken (p. 276). There are some uncanny parallels here to the Gnostic demiurge. Recall that it was the demiurge's insistence on his single nature that was later found to be in error, just as in Freud's own assessment of the ego. Further, it was the very existence of the demiurge's denial of other gods that simultaneously proved their existence, and in fact, it may have been the denial that allowed them to continue to work. Thus, both contrary realities exist "in the same breath," which is literally the case with the Gnostic creation of humans. The same notion is repeated in a later essay of Freud's (1940/1964), in which he writes of "two contrary and independent attitudes" (p. 204), which also "persist side by side throughout their lives without influencing each other" (p. 203).

In summary, Freud's splitting of the ego uniquely expresses the character of the Split Worlds myth, although the notion may not have been fully developed. Specifically, it expresses two halves of a single subject, both having conscious qualities and equally balanced, or symmetrical, but contradictory to each other. This is given by the simultaneous acknowledgment and disavowal of the same reality. In spite of this close proximity, the two sides persist in this state indefinitely, unable to affect the other. In other words, there is a lack of two-way causation, which leads to the condition of strong persistence. In the Split Worlds myth, this was associated with the long line of Tragic Transcenders.

The splitting of consciousness

Jung appears to have also dedicated attention to a similar psychological condition, although he never used Freud's terminology, as Freud focused on it after their separation. Rather, Jung's thoughts on the matter tend to aggregate around the more general term *dissociation*. However, the proposed conditions within this term are certainly not always clear. As with Freud, in which there are many types of splitting sometimes conflated, there are similarly many types of dissociation in Jung's writings. With Jung in general, it is often difficult to identify what kind of condition he is discussing, often due to his frequent use of metaphoric imagery. This is not necessarily due to intellectual laziness; he has at times stated his deliberate intentions to do so (Jung, 1950/1969, p. 13). Whether or not his reasons for this are justified, or whether it is effective, is beyond the scope of my argument, but it suffices to state that Jung's thoughts on such a topic requires significant additional interpretation. I am currently unaware of any attempt to tease out this particular subject from Jung's writings.

Some form of subjective-level splitting appears to be discussed in Jung's early work on schizophrenia. One such study was Jung's (1902/1983) evaluation of a classic case of the times, in which a patient was asked, "can you hear me?" The patient replies "No" (p. 53). This account is an effective presentation of vertical splitting, in that the subject both denies and acknowledges the question at the same time, in a single word. Or, as Freud would say, "in a single breath."

Jung describes two other cases with some similarities, this time focusing on the persistence of the condition. A young woman with "hysterical multiple personality" has become a variety of different personalities, who "keep to their respective roles and, if possible, do not bother each other" (Jung, 1939/1960, p. 235). Jung (1934/1969) elsewhere states that such "personality fragments undoubtedly have their own consciousness" (p. 97), and so it is given that consciousness itself can become split up. In another case, Jung (1928/1960) describes a hypothetical case in which a "subject has split into a plurality of subjects." This person may be a successful businessman, but an attack of paranoia reveals that he is actually "two egos" sharing one. "Neither of the two subjects can fully experience the other.... They know each other intimately, but they have no valid arguments against one another." Further, the subject can make multiple inconsistent statements in the same sentence, without any awareness that something is wrong. The subject becomes apathetic and "paralysed," on account of having "no central ego" (pp. 227–228).

In many of these accounts, there actually appears to be a conflation between vertical and horizontal splitting (Short, 2018, pp. 181–183), but these selected statements are still noted for their uncanny resemblances to Freud's formulation. Again, these would be the themes of multiple quasi-conscious fragments of a symmetrical nature, from which may issue a single, contradictory statement, and that of strong persistence, or lack of mutual causation. Jung may be also adding here the theme of the necessary lack of a central ego.

The same overall themes can be seen in Jung's later work, particularly those in which he turns his attention to the psychology of contemporary culture. As it turns out, I believe the subject of split consciousness may actually be best found in these writings. By contrast, the more traditional clinical material, involving analyst and patient, may not illustrate this particular dynamic very well.

The reason for this is given by Jung (1934/1970), as he describes two groups of people. Generally, there is the kind that comes in for personal analysis, versus those from the larger culture, that do not. It is this latter group that is described with characteristics resembling split consciousness, and their stories would not be portrayed in classical case studies.

Notably, both groups are understood to be affected by the unconscious, but the latter group may act in denial of this interaction. Thus, by their actions, they might simultaneously affirm and deny the existing of the unconscious, much like the Gnostic archons, "in one breath." Also, Jung (1934/1970) describes them not as one cohesive group, but actually consisting of many isolated, individual units. Each of these units act with a characteristic unfeeling toward the others, blaming them for all their own trouble, and expecting change to come from them. Therefore, overall, each of these units represents an element of consciousness, broken off from the other elements of consciousness, and the condition persists, due to this mutual and mistargeted blaming (pp. 138–139).

Jung draws on contemporary culture to provide specific examples of such an everlasting conflict. Crucially, Jung does not give any evidence that any of these split-off groups are more or less conscious than the other. In one essay, Jung (1961/1989) notes the conflicts between rationalism versus faith, with the latter including both Buddhists and Christians (pp. 256–262). Similarly, there is the conflict between the modern Church and State, each convinced of its own authority (p. 258). Jung also casts a wary eye at the conflict between West and East, who he says share the same intellectual assumptions. Further, none of the churches, in both regions, can change the course of politics (p. 265). Within the political sphere, both the Right and the Left employ equally one-sided rationalistic prejudices (p. 294).

However, perhaps the most dramatic split of this kind is that between faith and knowledge, between which an incommensurable "gulf" has opened up. Jung (1957/1970) describes this particular split in a way that concisely expresses many of the essential themes presented thus far, along with the proposed technical term.

> The rupture between faith and knowledge is a symptom of the *split consciousness* which is so characteristic of the mental disorder of our day. It is as if two different persons were making statements about the same thing, each from his own point of view... one person in two different frames of mind.
>
> (p. 285)

Also, without any intervention, perhaps from a third perspective, each is likely to continue obstinately in a state of mutual repression of the other, in a symmetrical manner (p. 286).

In summary so far, Jung's observations of contemporary cultural conflict are highly evocative of the phenomenon of splitting of consciousness, in a manner also consistent with Freud's splitting of the ego. The essential themes are, again, the symmetry of quasi-conscious entities, with none being primary, a lack of mutual causation, and occasioned by simultaneous contradiction. Fortunately, all of these relatively abstract notions can be effectively summarized by a single image, using Jung's metaphorical prose. "It is, indeed, the great trouble of our time that so many people exist whose right hand does not know what their left hand is doing" (Jung, 1961/1989, p. 193).

This notion of symmetry, or vertical splitting, is remarkably well captured with this image. This is a common expression in contemporary usage as well, commonly used to describe an overly complicated and ineffective bureaucratic system. Sometimes it is expressed in reverse, in both Jung's writings and in contemporary usage. That is, one can just as easily say that the left hand does not know what the right is doing, but the meaning of the phrase is the same. This would *not* be the case with the phrase "the mind does not know what the body is doing." Also, because the two hands are disconnected from each other, there is a lack of mutual causation, leading to strong persistence. Neither hand can effectively change the other, if it does not *know* what it is the other is doing.

I have now argued that the Cartesian Split is a vertical split, not a horizontal one, and this gives an entirely new way to apprehend it. Again, a horizontal split might be presented as the split between mind versus body, which is of course a common expression of the Cartesian Split. However, even mind versus body, *in this new context*, can also be interpreted as a vertical split, a splitting of consciousness. This can be seen simply from the notion that "body," from another perspective, *is itself an idea*. It is in fact a very well-developed idea, as shown in the Body as Machine metaphor above, used extensively in the highly *conscious* world of modern medicine. By contrast, the other idea, the idea of mind, is perhaps favored more by psychologists and philosophers. Therefore, the infamous Cartesian Split of mind versus body may not be about minds and bodies at all. Rather, it is about the *idea* of mind versus the *idea* of body. These two ideas are separate from each other, exactly as if one hand was unaware of the other. Given this, the Cartesian decapitated head takes on another meaning: There is no longer a central head that might possibly connect the two.

Interestingly, this interpretation I am now applying relates well with the general usage of the word "split." In general, it seems that we almost always use this term to denote a nearly symmetrical divide. For example, to share a payment, we split the difference into two equal halves. A split second means only smaller, equivalent bits of sub-seconds. We also use it in terms related to consciousness. A split jury is perfectly balanced, an equal number of guilty and not guilty votes. Similarly, a boxing match is left without a clear winner if the judges give a split decision. These are examples of conscious statements of generally equal value, and so no clear decision can be made. Similar usage is found in descriptions of things. A computer display can go into split-screen mode, to show you two equally important windows of knowledge. We often say we have a splitting headache, which is all in the head, but we never have a splitting body ache, even with the flu. Finally, when we think too much, we are splitting hairs, which of course are all on the head. These last two examples are strikingly consistent with the theme of Over-rationality.

After Jung provides the image of disconnected hands, he immediately provides another important insight. Jung (1961/1989) states that this condition is not a recent development, nor unique to the Christian world, but rather, it is "the symptom of a general unconsciousness that is the heritage of all mankind" (p. 193). In other words, it is archetypal. The underlying archetype of the Cartesian Split complex can now be named, which follows naturally from the image of disconnected hands. The split-off hands still function, but in an isolated existence, unaware of each other, and therefore unable to affect the other. This is the archetype of *dismemberment*.

However, one further qualification to this is necessary. Properly speaking, this notion is only one half of the archetype. It is a *tragic* dismemberment, one that must be undone. There are many creation myths in which a god is dismembered, and this is seen as necessary for human life, such as with Osiris, Tiamet, and Dionysus. The remnants of divinity, scattered throughout the world, can still bring life. By contrast, when humans are dismembered by a god, this is a terrible tragedy, and only brings death. This kind of dismemberment *must be undone* for new life to occur. In short, a god can handle dismemberment, but a human cannot.

Modern dismemberment

In summary so far, the Cartesian Split complex is modern myth in disguise, a myth that suggests that something has gone tragically wrong with the creation of consciousness. In most world mythologies, the original creation of consciousness is a positive event, symbolized by an original cosmic separation. There is no such myth for us in modern times. Rather, we seem to now be living in a myth in which separations must be mended. However, the separation that must be mended is not the original one, it is a secondary separation that has occurred within consciousness itself. This has divided humanity right down the middle, just as the vengeful Zeus did eons ago, with his fearsome thunderbolts from heaven. He split Male from Female, and warned if humans were to keep acting up, he would do it again. This dirty deed may have been left up to his modern incarnation, the villainous Descartes, who has truly done it again, this time splitting Left from Right, also in a top-down manner. Only this Split is not from heaven, but from his thinking, the notorious *Meditations*. Now, we are truly dismembered, feckless, each of us hopping around on only one leg.

This new expression of dismemberment can now be used to revisit the other themes in the review of abstracts. Many of these themes were originally presented in a manner in which they seemed incoherent, perhaps the result of simply poor scholarship. Now, they can all be seen as integrally related, as an especially poignant expression of psychic dismemberment, or split consciousness.

The Body as Machine metaphor can be instantly recognized as such. There is strong sympathy for the critique of this idea. One looks at their own hand, and, although it moves, the textbooks say it is nothing more than a collection of bones, muscles, and tendons, obeying electrical impulses. The tragedy of this conception is that one does not *feel* the hand as part of one's own essence, from the inside out. In this way, it might as well be a dismembered hand.

Another prominent theme was Ecological Crisis, and this can be understood more easily if ecology is not understood literally as the physical environment, but rather as symbolic of the psychical environment. Both Freud and Jung liberally employed topographical models of the psyche, consisting of various layers, with images taken from the natural world. Indeed, Jung even considered himself an archaeologist of the soul and frequently compared the deep psyche to nature. Naturally, a tragic dismemberment of the environment of the psyche is an ecological disaster that needs attention.

Several authors lamented Cartesian influence as that of holding back artistic expression, and even in preventing progresses in the sciences. In other words, neither the hand of the arts nor the hand of the sciences can affect the other, and so nothing changes. There is no new creation, no new life, because no new symbols are created. Etymologically, the meaning of the word *symbol* is "throwing together," and so a tragic dismemberment is what prevents this from occurring. It is as if the two dismembered hands just keep switching sides, but remain disconnected, unable to yield any productive work.

Finally, with the image of dismemberment, the theme of Charged Images takes on fresh new meaning. Earlier, I argued this was simply indicative of a complex in general, to the extent that all complexes are emotionally charged. But there is something unique with all the gruesome scenes of dismemberment that accompany the Cartesian Split. We have seen mothers decapitating her children, humans ripped apart and turned to monsters, and souls rent into dread chasms, leaving behind only the haunting of a disembodied ghost. In comparison, Freud says there is a hidden rift in the ego, which "never heals," and Jung (1957/1970) talks of a "boundary line bristling with barbed wire [that] runs through the psyche of modern man, no matter on which side he lives" (p. 280).

It is with these latter reflections that the overall feeling of the Cartesian Split complex is unique. All complexes are emotional, but this one seems to carry a significant amount of additional weight. These new images, that of dismemberment, ecological disaster, decapitations, and dread chasms, *are not just simply emotional.* Rather, it is as if they were uniquely intended to evoke in us the deepest kind of empathic reaction. Even the most unfeeling rationalist could only react to these images in horror. If we fully take them in, they can strike us to the core, down to bone and sinew. Some kind of internal tragedy has occurred, and this now demands our fullest attention.

References

Baker, G. P., & Morris, K. J. (2002). *Descartes' dualism.* London, UK: Routledge.

Berman, M. (1981). *The reenchantment of the world.* Ithaca, NY: Cornell University Press.

Brook, J. A. (1992). Freud and splitting. *International Review of Psycho-Analysis, 19,* 335–350.

Campbell, J. (1983). *Historical atlas of world mythology.* New York, NY: Harper & Row.

Edinger, E. F. (1984). *The creation of consciousness: Jung's myth for modern man.* Toronto, Canada: Inner City Books.

Erlanger, O., & Govela, L. O. (2018, November 27). The origins of Silicon Valley's garage myth. Retrieved October 20, 2019, from Fast Company website: https://www.fastcompany.com/90270226/the-origins-of-silicon-valleys-garage-myth

Freud, S. (1964). An outline of psycho-analysis. In J. Strachey (Ed.), *Moses and monotheism: An outline of psycho-analysis and other works* (pp. 141–208). London, UK: Hogarth Press. (Original work published 1940)

Freud, S. (1964). Splitting of the ego in the process of defence. In J. Strachey (Ed.), *Moses and monotheism: An outline of psycho-analysis and other works* (pp. 271–278). London, UK: Hogarth Press. (Original work published 1938)

Hoeller, S. A. (1982). *The gnostic Jung and the seven sermons to the dead* (1st ed.). Wheaton, IL: Theosophical Pub. House.

Jacobi, J. (1968). *The psychology of C. G. Jung: An introduction with illustrations.* New Haven, CT: Yale University Press.

Jung, C. G. (1960). Mental disease and the psyche. In R. F. C. Hull (Trans.), *The collected works of C. G. Jung* (Vol. 3, pp. 226–230). Princeton, NJ: Princeton University Press. (Original work published 1928)

Jung, C. G. (1960). On the psychogenesis of schizophrenia. In R. F. C. Hull (Trans.), *The collected works of C. G. Jung* (Vol. 3, pp. 233–249). Princeton, NJ: Princeton University Press. (Original work published 1939)

Jung, C. G. (1969). A review of the complex theory. In R. F. C. Hull (Trans.), *The collected works of C. G. Jung* (Vol. 8, pp. 92–104). Princeton, NJ: Princeton University Press. (Original work published 1934)

Jung, C. G. (1969). *Aion: Researches into the phenomenology of the self* (R. F. C. Hull, Trans.). Princeton, NJ: Princeton University Press. (Original work published 1950)

Jung, C. G. (1969). The transcendent function. In R. F. C. Hull (Trans.), *The collected works of C. G. Jung* (Vol. 8, pp. 67–91). Princeton, NJ: Princeton University Press. (Original work published 1928)

Jung, C. G. (1970). The meaning of psychology for modern man. In R. F. C. Hull (Trans.), *The collected works of C. G. Jung* (Vol. 10, pp. 134–156). Princeton, NJ: Princeton University Press. (Original work published 1934)

Jung, C. G. (1970). The role of the unconscious. In R. F. C. Hull (Trans.), *The collected works of C. G. Jung* (Vol. 10, pp. 3–28). Princeton, NJ: Princeton University Press. (Original work published 1918)

Jung, C. G. (1970). The undiscovered self. In R. F. C. Hull (Trans.), *The collected works of C. G. Jung* (Vol. 10, pp. 245–305). Princeton, NJ: Princeton University Press. (Original work published 1957)

Jung, C. G. (1983). On the psychology and pathology of so-called occult phenomena. In R. F. C. Hull (Trans.), *The collected works of C. G. Jung* (Vol. 1, pp. 3–88). Princeton, NJ: Princeton University Press. (Original work published 1902)

Jung, C. G. (1989). Symbols and the interpretation of dreams. In R. F. C. Hull (Trans.), *The collected works of C. G. Jung* (Vol. 18, pp. 183–264). Princeton, NJ: Princeton University Press. (Original work published 1961)

Jung, C. G., & Jaffé, A. (1989). *Memories, dreams, reflections* (Rev. ed). New York, NY: Vintage Books.

Kelso, C. (2015, February 10). Reuniting the apparent mind/body split. Retrieved February 17, 2019, from The Deepest Peace website: https://thedeepestpeace.com/2015/02/10/reuniting-the-apparent-mindbody-split/#more-413

Maguire, R. (1997). "Proofs of God's existence:" Walker Percy, Jacques Maritain, and the problem of the symbol in the moviegoer. *Logos: A Journal of Catholic Thought and Culture, 1*(3), 69–79. doi: 10.1353/log.1997.0018

Meyer, M. (Ed.). (2007). *The Nag Hammadi scriptures.* San Francisco, CA: HarperSanFrancisco.

Pether, P. (1999). On foreign ground: Grand narratives, situated specificities, and the praxis of critical theory and law. *Law and Critique, 10*(3), 211–236. Retrieved from eoah: https://link.springer.com/article/10.1023/A:1008942114765.

Short, B. (2018). *The depths of the Cartesian split: A hidden myth in modern psychology* (Doctoral dissertation). Pacifica Graduate Institute. (10822143).

Spuybroek, L. (1999). The Cartesian split. *ANY: Architecture New York,* 24, 13–13. Retrieved from JSTOR: https://www.jstor.org/stable/i40087763.

von Franz, M.-L. (1972). *Patterns of creativity mirrored in creation myths.* Dallas, TX: Spring.

Chapter 7

Cultural memories

From the perspective I have constructed, the Cartesian Split has less to do with the history of philosophy and more to do with the current nature of collective consciousness. The overall tone of the discussion is indicative of a complex, and the symbolic material embedded in it suggests that consciousness has somehow become split, fragmented, dismembered. It is important to note that the nature of this split is not between consciousness and anything else. Rather, the split is within consciousness itself. The right hand does not know what the left hand is doing, nor does the left hand know of the right. And yet, they live on, although in seemingly separate existences. Perhaps they interact, but not really, as they are unable to meaningfully affect each other. At the individual level, this is characterized by a contradiction within the subject, and given by a simultaneous acknowledgment and disavowal of a single object. Collectively, it can be seen in cultural fragmentation, in which there is a strong persistence of divisive conflict, in which no one group is more or less conscious than the others. If this is an accurate assessment, then the phenomenon needs to be pulled away from the rote history of philosophy and placed against a wider context. This is the goal of this chapter.

In the case of Ash, this would be the moment where a different narrative is constructed. The initial sessions were used to differentiate the myth from mundane reality. That is, the fantastic story of Rand was distinguished from the actual Rand, and Ash was included in this slow, painstaking effort. Once this was done, an interpretation was made privately, using the amplifications from other mythic stories. Now that Ash can understand that the story is not really about Rand, Ash is seeking to understand the true origins of this story. In other words, what events that actually happened may have laid the foundations for this present struggle? This requires a process of self-inquiry, a critical venture of self-knowledge. What is truly different about Ash that is different from the others? Why is Ash struggling with this alone, and what does it mean? Ash may ask: Who am I really, and what exactly am I trying to work out?

The Anglo-split

I have thus far explored the archetypal basis of the phenomenon, which indicates that the underlying psychological condition is universal. However, archetypes are always expressed in the form of complexes, which are uniquely located in specific cultural conditions, and this is what makes the myth of the Cartesian Split unique. In this instance, the initial story was presented in terms of the whole Western world, whose entire philosophical underpinnings have now come into question. However, the conditions of this particular story can now be made more specific than this.

The prominent philosophical arguments, those that formed the basis of my study, already pointed in this direction. Lovejoy (1955) celebrated the Great Revolt not across Europe, but only in the "English-speaking part of the world" (p. 1). Baker and Morris (2002) specifically locate their Cartesian Legend, or the basic Two-Worlds view, in Anglo-American philosophers (p. x). Similarly, Cottingham (1998) notes specific problems of misunderstanding on the subject only in Anglophone philosophers (p. 19). Further, Wilson (1993) is suspicious of existing commentary on Descartes, "especially those writing in English" (p. vii). Finally, Graffman (2017) documents an article surveying all possible reactions to "the Cartesian gap," and this list is heavily Anglophone (p. 148). Overall, these surprisingly specific localizations have only been observed within the field of academic philosophy.

In my study, I have expanded the scope to other fields, from which I have derived the larger Split Worlds myth. However, my review of such commentary has mostly confirmed this original localization. For example, the most vociferous critiques I have found were from Capra and Hillman, both of whom studied and wrote in English. Capra, although born and educated in Austria, did his history of science work in America, at which time he became strongly interested in Descartes. Hillman is American by birth. By contrast, the Swiss Jung, writing in German, was noted to be unusually quiet on the subject. Also, it is worth noting that I did most of my original research without paying direct attention to this localization. In other words, I seem to have independently corroborated it, and from within a much larger review of material.

Of course, the notion of a dramatic psychological split can be related to similar notions found outside of Anglophone sources. Most notably, a parallel can be drawn to Kant's seeming impassable divide between the subject and the thing-in-itself. The field of phenomenology, featuring the contributions of Husserl, Merleau-Ponty, Sartre, and Heidegger, can all be seen as acting in response to this divide. However, my study has been focused on the particularly vehement, mythological reactions to a specific caricature of Descartes, and these subjects are generally lacking in this. Heidegger and Merleau-Ponty are critical of Descartes, but no more than is necessary to advance their own arguments. Husserl is openly appreciative of him. Further, upon inspection, all of these theorists seem to be really concerned with the divide between the subject and reality, and not within the subject itself, as in the case with split consciousness.

Even theorists who might be considered to be dealing with split consciousness, do not invoke Descartes' name, if they are not writing in English. Max Weber, in his landmark *Science as a Vocation,* invokes a Split Worlds image remarkably similar to Jung's. However, the non-English Weber, like the non-English Jung, does not blame Descartes, even though the description is strongly evocative of the Split Worlds. Weber (1946) writes of "the various value spheres of the world (that) stand in irreconcilable conflict with each other" (p. 144), and that "the tension between the value-spheres of 'science' and the sphere of 'the holy' is unbridgeable" (p. 151). In this case, unbridgeable "spheres" seem to translate directly to Cartesian split "worlds," and yet, Weber does not describe them as such.

Additionally, it has been suggested that the affected culture is not necessarily Anglophone in general, but specifically Anglophone scholars, and there is good reason for this. Outside of academia, there is likely only a superficial awareness of Descartes. If he is even known, he is probably known only for "I think, therefore I am," and not for any kind of infamous split. Naturally, if one were to interrogate a nonacademic on some of the mind-body problems raised by Descartes, there would surely be an answer involving some problematic assumptions. However, the problem would only be a real concern for the academic; the subject would likely go on with their day completely unperturbed, whereas the academic would feel compelled to write a critique, bemoaning the continued influence of Cartesian thought. However, even this evaluation is questionable. Hodge (2008) argues that scholars often uncritically assume that "folk psychology" is permeated with Cartesian dualism, but that this claim does not hold up to the evidence. In any case, even though the discussion is limited to scholars, the academic community cannot possibly be considered as entirely separate from its broader cultural matrix. It is enough for now to suggest that the academic community is an abstracted voice of this particular cultural complex, expressed in scholarly terms. Perhaps it is in academia where the complex is best expressed and developed, and following which, may be re-integrated back into the larger culture.

The obvious question is then, what is unique to Anglophone culture that would predispose it to this voice, featuring such complex-ridden arguments? What are the deeper cultural roots that may be informing it, and what are its origins? The remainder of this chapter will attempt to answer these questions.

It might go without saying that such an inquiry is riddled with uncommon difficulty. It is difficult enough to presume a generally valid characterization of the entirety of Anglophone culture, let alone that of viewing it in terms of my working interpretation, that of split consciousness, which is itself somewhat tentative. Further, the broader question is well outside of my field of expertise, involving a myriad of cultural, social, and historical factors, that cannot possibly be fully or properly considered in this work. Nonetheless, the narrative I have constructed seems to naturally invite such questions, and so an attempt must be made.

Anamnesis

The first attempt toward this goal is to consider the historical aspect of the myth under study. Even though it ultimately concerns the nature of present-day consciousness, its excessive interest in deep philosophical history is undeniable. The myth is impressively multifaceted, but it does feature one strongly consistent narrative: Something bad happened at the beginning of the modern age. Overall, I have interpreted this as being symbolic of the creation of consciousness, which is timeless, but it need not be entirely symbolic. For Jung, a symbol is always a "best possible expression" of something unknown, and therefore, if it strongly and consistently indicates a specific point in time, it behooves at least a consideration that this one aspect is factual. Combined with the above-noted Anglophone culture, the best approach would then be to recall significant cultural events in the late medieval period, on the British Isles.

A new look at olde times

The most natural events to focus on would then be the English Renaissance and Reformation, in the late 16th century. Again, there has been voluminous research on this topic, and it is far beyond the scope of this work to cover it all. However, even a cursory review of sources indicates that this was indeed a highly tumultuous period, one that might be conducive to the formation of a cultural complex. The conventional narrative is that the Renaissance, Reformation, and subsequent Scientific Enlightenment was a time of beneficent progress, gradually displacing the darkness and superstitions of the Middle Ages. However, historian Trevor-Roper (1999) notes that each of these three developments was accompanied by a significant amount of tragedy. Specifically, the witch-craze of the 16th and 17th centuries is a sobering reminder that the wheels of progress sometimes move backward. Simply put, there was no witch-craze in "the Dark Age" (pp. 83–84).

Historians such as Duffy, Scarisbrick, and Haigh suggest that the real history is even darker, focusing on the tragic acts of suppression that accompanied the Reformation under Henry VIII. This has earned them the somewhat dubious distinction of "revisionist" historians (Johnson, 1997, paras. 1–4). Of these, Duffy deserves special mention, particularly for his *The Stripping of the Altars*, a master inventory of traumatic losses suffered by the English laity during the Reformation. In order for Protestantism to prosper, significant Catholic heritage had to be destroyed, and this amounted to a great loss. Regardless of the merits of this work, the author's own evaluation of it places it firmly in the territory of the Anglophone Cartesian Split complex. Duffy (2005) argues that the Reformation amounted to a "great cultural hiatus, which had dug a ditch, deep and dividing, between the English people and their past." A thousand years of rich history was not just lost but became utterly unknown, an "alien territory, the dark ages of 'popery'" (p. xiv).

Also deserving of special mention is Selwood, an admirer of Duffy, and who adds a further twist to this newly evident tragedy. Selwood (2015) argues that the conventional narrative of progress and liberation is not just wrong, but devious. It is argued to be nothing but propaganda, intentionally fabricated by the reformers for their own political purposes. According to this view, the Tudors wanted even more power, and to do so, they had to violently suppress the practices of peaceful English Catholics, who mostly did not want change.

Again, from my limited position, I cannot take a firm position in this debate, but from a depth psychological perspective, something certainly appears to be developing in this new look at a fundamental period of English history. Even if not a single fact were produced that supported this revisionist view, the mere presence of a desire to look for them is psychologically significant. It is also worth noting that the "revisionist" view for dedicated scholars of English history is almost taken as axiomatic by those outside the field. Bordo, it is to be recalled, reads Descartes as an expression of a pathology of modernism, the loss of the "organic female universe." The tragic nature of this background is generally pre-supposed. Therefore, the overall situation is befitting of a cultural complex, with such a wide polarization of views across disparate disciplines.

Regardless, there can be no doubt that certain lines of cultural fragmentation appeared during this time. It must be significant that the Reformation was followed by the violent Puritan Revolution, a Counter-Reformation, and three civil wars. The residual tension between Irish Catholics and Protestants today would be only one small example of the continued presence of these lines of fragmentation. The exact nature of English culture before the Reformation may be debated, but it can at least be described in singular terms, that of being mostly Catholic, with its rulers aligned with Rome. Such a singular characterization is of course much less likely to be found today.

Overall, the various difficulties of this approach may be mitigated by maintaining the symbolic approach, which I have used throughout this study. As I have stated, the nature of consciousness is best expressed in symbolic form, and this would also apply to cultural expressions of its pathology. In this case, I would then turn to prominent cultural art forms during this time, in order to explore possible indications of the formation of split consciousness. This effort is assisted by noting the preferred archetypal expression of this condition, that of dismemberment.

Therefore, a starting assumption for this investigation would be the following: The Cartesian Split complex has roots in an unconscious Anglophone cultural memory, resulting from a tragic Reformation, which coincided with an onset of cultural fragmentation and symbolized by human dismemberment. If this supposition were to have any validity at all, there would then be dramatic themes of dismemberment featured in the most prominent cultural art forms of the day.

Dismemberment on stage

Margaret Owens is a professor of English who specializes in early modern literature and has written a monograph on exactly this topic. While researching acts of violence in the *Annals of English Drama 975–1700*, Owens (2005) made a surprising discovery, that "severed heads and dismembered body parts turn up with remarkable frequency in late medieval and Renaissance drama" (p. 13).

Owens (2005) notes that such scenes are uniquely powerful and cannot be understood simply as general dramatic provocation. Something about images of dismemberment strikes a unique chord in us, one that carries a specific set of associations, perhaps reminding us of our deepest vulnerabilities. Owens employs a psychoanalytic approach and interprets images of the body as a metaphor for the essence of the individual. She also follows Lacan's notion of the "fragilized ego," by which it is meant that we are inherently fragile, at the deepest level of our identity. Dismemberment in this context is therefore a powerful expression of subjective fragility, or in other words, the possibility of split consciousness. Further, such a visual metaphor can act at both the individual and cultural levels, and there is something about it that seems "timeless," "almost ubiquitous," and valid for many cultures (pp. 11–12). In other words, it is archetypal. Overall, these assumptions are consistent with my interpretation of split consciousness, its preferred modes of expression, and its archetypal roots.

Not surprisingly, Owens (2005) appears to be sympathetic to the revisionist view of English Reformation history. Although the break with Rome must have produced some feelings of liberation, such new-found freedom must have also been accompanied by feelings of anxiety (pp. 19–20). In general, her "study rests on the assumption that Protestant Reformation figured as a traumatic rupture in sixteenth-century English culture." Although Owens admits that the word "trauma" might be debatable, she maintains that "there is no disputing the fact that the Reformation affected every aspect of the nation's social fabric." The image that readily comes to mind for her is the burning of heretics, by both Protestant and Catholic regimes (p. 22). In summary, the Reformation can certainly be seen as conducive toward the formation of a cultural complex.

However, before delving into the specifics of such cultural events, it is best to begin with the symbolic images that typically accompany them. In any case, whatever the nature of individual or cultural fragmentation that was occurring at the time, surely the highly popular stage play would serve as a reliable symbolic testimony. In support of this, Owens does in fact present an intriguing development in the nature of theatric dismemberment, in the plays of this period.

The sudden shift

Owens (2005) emphasizes that the theme of dismemberment did not just suddenly appear. Rather, it was a well-developed thematic element, one that appeared prominently and regularly for centuries before the Reformation, mostly in what is known as the saint plays. What is significant for the time of the Reformation is the transformation, of both the manifest content and its perceived meaning. In the saint plays of the prior period, various saints were often graphically shown to be tortured, dismembered, and eventually killed, usually through decapitation. However, crucially, this was likely understood by audiences in mostly positive terms. The saint was the hero of the play, who demonstrated spiritual strength through his or her ability to withstand torture. In fact, the more gruesome the violence, the more heroic the saint. Such superhuman ability was understood in terms of the imitation of Christ, and this had a therapeutic effect on the audience (pp. 18–19). In other words, the saint plays served to maintain and communicate orthodox doctrine regarding personal salvation. A lay individual may have been liable to suffering and fragmentation, but from the continued demonstrations of the saints, a wholesome sense of identity could be restored. In short, scenes of dismemberment were fully contained within Catholic dogma and carried with them a single, positive message.

Owens's overall thesis rests on the observation that scenes of dismemberment in post-Reformation plays are drastically different, indicating that this message was significantly altered by the events of the Reformation. She traces this overall development through a detailed study of many plays, focusing on R.B.'s *Apius and Virginia*, Shakespeare's *2 Henry VI*, and finally Marlowe's *Dr. Faustus*. All of these have unusually violent or disproportionate scenes of dismemberment, with potentially different meanings, which represents a significant shift away from the traditional saint plays. I cannot review all the arguments for this development, but for the sake of economy, I can present those in *Dr. Faustus*, given that it can be seen to encapsulate most of this progression. This play certainly has an impressive inventory of scenes of explicit dismemberment, with additional implicit references, which run throughout the entire play.

The story begins with Faustus, a scholar and doctor who came from lowly origins but quickly ascended to prominence. However, he is dissatisfied with the ultimate aim of all conventional studies, so he turns to the dark arts of necromancy. He makes a pact with Mephistophilis, to have extraordinary power and knowledge for 24 years, at the end of which time Lucifer will claim him for eternity. This time is somewhat wasted, however, as his powers are spent on gaining only modest increases in knowledge. Mephistophilis is reticent when Faustus comes to the most important questions. Also, although he gains various physical powers, he generally only uses them to perform impish tricks on others. Also, throughout the play, Faustus agonizes with internal doubt over his decision, wavering violently back and forth between two states. Either he marvels over his wondrous talents, or he falls into deep despair over his inevitable damnation. He also wavers back and forth between spiritual inclinations and general hedonism.

Three scenes in particular feature graphic dismemberment. Faustus tricks one character into playing Actaeon, which puts him in danger of being ravaged by hunting dogs. But his victims regroup, with a plot to cut off Faustus's head and to further dismember him. They strike the blow, but Faustus heals instantly, a power he gained from his pact with Mephistophilis. Later, his leg is pulled off and carried away, but this also later heals (Owens, 2005, pp. 227–228). In the final scene, when his time is up, Mephistophilis comes for his soul and tears him to pieces. Witnesses note that the shrieks and cries from that dreadful night were the worst since the dawn of creation. Playgoers were likely treated with a horrifying display of bloody fragments, which this time, of course, do not heal (pp. 228, 249).

From this, it is already quite obvious that this is no traditional saint play, the likes of which were common before the Reformation. Indeed, Faustus is almost the antithesis of a saint. He chooses the Devil over God, is hedonistic and greedy, displays little strength of conviction, and dies ingloriously in the end, rather than heroically (Owens, 2005, p. 242). And yet, at the same time, the overall structural pattern is the same: The main character suffers bodily dismemberment but is unaffected. Also, he stays the course and finally meets a dramatic ending. And so, the inversion is at the same time a restatement, although in a dramatically different form (p. 243).

What is most different is that, in a short period of time, the venerated saint had become a damned fool. Rather than being a martyr, setting a positive example, Faustus's story seems a senseless tragedy. The violence, once religiously meaningful, has now become disturbing, or perhaps even comical. The saint, once the object of the highest possible respect, has become an object of pity.

Also, Owens (2005) notes that the playhouse itself was transformed at this time. What once was an officially sanctioned vehicle of the church's message, was now placed in the hands of more commercial interests. This would have the effect of the people beginning to doubt and mistrust the playhouses (p. 19). This can be compared to how the Gnostics began to doubt and mistrust their rulers. But perhaps simple doubt is preferable to fear and terror. At one point during the transformation of the saint play, Henry VIII attended a play in which he himself was portrayed as the beheader of the saint. The frightful part is that this coincided with a certain "slippage" from the fanciful to the literal, as it turns out that the king had ordered an actual beheading only one day earlier, executing a Catholic bishop who had questioned the king's legitimacy (pp. 44–46). Further, there may have been a certain sick joy in all this. According to one blogger, "Henry VIII loved separating folks from the Earth almost as much as he loved separating the Church of England from the Roman Catholics" (Richard, 2019, para. 2).

The splitting of ritual

It is this sudden shift in the dramatic enactment of bodily dismemberment, along with an increased fascination with it, that Owens finds to be culturally significant. Specifically, she argues it was intimately bound up with the highly charged religious disputes of the Reformation, occurring at the same time. To highlight the nature of this relationship, Owens (2005) focuses on the highly contentious issue of transubstantiation, the rejection of which might be labeled "the axis of the Reformist program" (p. 18).

Transubstantiation is an idea almost alien to modern sensibilities, yet it occupied a central position in pre-Reformation society. This was the belief, carefully enacted in the ritual of the Catholic Eucharist, or communion, that the bread and wine are physically transformed into the blood and flesh of Christ. Thus, upon eating and drinking, the participant was able to take part in the immediate salvific presence of the body of Christ. The body of the sinner and the body of Savior were reconciled, physically and immediately (Owens, 2005, p. 18). It is important to note that the manifest qualities of the bread and wine were understood not to change. The perceived sensations of taste, that of familiar bread and wine, was unchanged. However, the substance in which those qualities inhered did change, from bread to flesh, hence the term *transubstantiation*. This transformation was understood to be a miracle, a most holy sacrament, and administered only by an elect clergy.

However, the Protestants made a pointed rejection of this belief. The bread and wine were now argued not to be physically changed, and Owens (2005) believes that this rejection resulted in a profound loss. Although seemingly more rational, the possibility of immediate physical experience with the divine was now precluded. It was now only possible in the distant past when Christ literally walked the earth (pp. 17–18). Personal experience was still emphasized, but the focus of attention was now toward the close reading of scripture. The ritual of communion was maintained, but Christ's immediate presence is missing. Rather, the ritual was performed only "in remembrance of me," that is, of Christ's original last supper, which only happened once in history. Therefore, reconciliation depended solely on the ability to make the symbolic link between present bread and historical flesh, in the mind.

Owens (2005) states that the original unquestioned belief in transubstantiation was intimately bound up with the traditional saint plays, which were common before the Reformation. When a saint was dismembered on stage, the audience member could understand it in terms of Christ's dismemberment. That same person would then have been able to go to mass the very same day, and experience Christ's body and blood, directly, physically, and immediately. More importantly, the sense of individual integrity and personal wholeness was able to be restored. Christ was not just remembered from a historical memory, but physically re-*membered*, in the individual, in the present moment. Fundamentally, there was the belief that "the human body could provide access to the sacred" (pp. 17–18).

This sense of immediate physical reconciliation was seemingly lost as a result of the Reformation, and this loss is argued to be reflected by the shift of dismemberment on stage. However, such a loss need not be seen in wholly negative terms. Owens (2005) refers to this kind of evaluation as the "lapsarian" view, in which the Middle Ages are seen as a period of unbroken, organic wholeness, lost irrevocably and tragically by the Reformation. However, Owens takes care to avoid a firm commitment to this view. She argues simply that before the Reformation, the meaning of dismemberment was effectively contained in prevailing dogma; she does not insist on the value of that containment. She also notes that this containment showed ample signs of failure long before the Reformation (p. 19).

Surely, the Reformers must have had valid complaints against the orthodoxy, including valid arguments against the doctrine of transubstantiation. Although this ritual had the advantage of being physically real and present, it was also governed over wholly by priests, who may have abused such privilege (Owens, 2005, p. 55). The individual may have had access to the sacred through their body, but this access was still governed over by external authorities. You could not take mass at home. The Reformation aimed for an individual to have a personal experience of God, without the need for any intermediary, who might not be able to be trusted.

The Protestant reformers had many other critiques on their agenda. In general, they were highly suspicious of any claim of present-day miracles, specifically those that were governed over by the clergy. One of their favorite rhetorical tactics was to suggest that the entire enactment of the mass was nothing more than an elaborate theatrical performance, but with the intent to deceive. The miracles of the sacraments were exposed as mere trickery, in order to dupe the people into following the program. The Protestant argument was therefore a plea for a kind of rationalism. The priest, it was said, could not actually transform bread into flesh, nor bless ordinary water into holy water (Owens, 2005, pp. 235–236). Bread was bread and water was water. Physical miracles were only able to be performed once in history, by one person, Christ alone. In fact, the clergy could now be considered the true blasphemers for trying to replicate them. The best miracle one could hope for in the present came from the study of scripture, and through the personal acceptance of Christ by faith.

Surely, there must have been some strong resistance to this radically new set of beliefs. The mere existence of the Counter-Reformation is evidence enough of that. Overall, it is easy to imagine a deep rift forming in the overall social fabric. On one hand, there were the Reformers, who probably had valid complaints against a corrupt and devious orthodoxy, along with strong appeals to common sense, and increased individual freedom. On the other hand, there were the Catholics, who could have insisted that only their officially sanctioned rituals provided immediate and physical religious experience, along with the security of tradition. To stray from this aura of protection was to invite certain damnation.

The splitting of the play

Dr. Faustus was being performed at exactly the same time as this debate was raging among the public, and therefore can be seen as a microcosm of the Reformation debate. Not too surprisingly, Owens (2005) notes that there are two different possible interpretations of the play, and these have survived to the present day. On one hand, there is the "doctrinal" interpretation, in which the play reflects the Catholic orthodoxy's admonition against the occult, against leaving the protection of the church and their officially sanctioned rituals. Others have taken up the "heterodox" interpretation, in which the same admonition is essentially mocked, and so earthly experience is not a heresy, but encouraged. It therefore contains a hidden message that sanctions leaving the church (p. 232).

Historically, it can be imagined that a Catholic and a Protestant could have attended the exact same performance of this play, and yet walk away with two entirely different interpretations about what they just saw. A Catholic viewer may have appreciated the lesson of this tragedy: Faustus is damned to hell for outright heresy, and for using his devilish powers for selfish, hedonistic concerns. He is also blasphemous for attempting the sacred miracles himself. By contrast, a Protestant might have seen the same production as a comical farce, having already formed the same opinion of the stage-magic of the mass. Or, the Protestant may also have witnessed the lesson of blasphemy, but flipped around.

This would have been easy for a Protestant viewer to see, as trickery was well known as a theatric device. The scenes of miraculous dismemberment in plays were performed using various stage tricks, such as fake heads and other illusions. In the case of the play, of course, everyone knew that the actor's head was not really being cut off. The actors were highly trained professionals who were able to manipulate devices in order to produce the illusion. Similarly, the Reformers viewed the rituals performed in the mass with equal suspicion. The bread was not really being transformed, this was argued to be a mere theatrical trick, performed by a highly trained clergy, who knew how to manipulate the articles of the sacrament, in order to deceive. And so, in this view, Faustus is indeed damned as a blasphemer, only now he is the representative of the corrupt orthodox. Only the Protestant, who rejected the orthodox rituals altogether, could be safe from this deception. No doubt they would have enjoyed the image of the venerable saint turned upside-down, into an object of ridicule.

Either way, for both the Catholic and the Protestant, Faustus gets what he deserved, and so it is easy to see why the play was so popular. This is especially true when considering cultural psychology. It is always a popular message to the people when you get to blame "the others," and enjoy their eventual comeuppance. It is even more popular when you can use the same message to appeal to both audiences at the same time.

However, there may have also been a sense of anxiety drawing them to the performances. In spite of perhaps the occasional laugh, the visuals alone would have been enough to produce a certain sense of anxiety and must have been compounded by the attendant religious implications. Specifically, there were two radically different ways to understand the meaning of the symbolism on stage, in terms of the original ritual. Accordingly, there was now a very high stake made on which interpretation to follow, upon which rested *nothing less that the fate of the soul.* It would be very unwise to underestimate the importance of this to a late medieval person.

Further, this may have been a problem not only for the day of reckoning but also for the present. Again, rituals provide for immediate salvation, felt in flesh and bone. An audience member may have no longer been certain as to how to understand the constitution of their own body and its relationship to the sacred. By extension, this could manifest in various painful doubts concerning the possibility of wholeness and of secure identity, in the present moment.

Where once the body provided immediate, physical access to the sacred, there was now a political battleground, between rival forces, each with compelling arguments. One side said we can provide it through our ritual, through your body. The other side said it happens through our interpretations, through your mind. Where once the body-mind was made whole through the miracle of transubstantiation, there was now only doubt. In Owens's (2005) words, the body's own "signifying capacities were malleable and open to dispute." Also, with the loss of the saints, who once visually demonstrated the way of the miracle, the dispute was now left open to the playhouses, or the "hands of corrupt and tyrannical forces" (p. 23).

The anxiety this would have produced must have been terrific, and this is matched only by the excessive spectacle of Faustus's demise. Owens (2005) argues that it was likely that Faustus's bloody remains were shown in graphic detail. The sourcebook of the play features brains on walls, eyes and teeth scattered, and other parts strewn on dung heaps (p. 249). This could have been a highly appropriate reflection of an audience member's own dueling anxieties, concerning the nature of the body, and the fate of their soul. It is not too daring to suggest that this anxiety has been left unresolved.

The splitting of cultural consciousness

Such unresolved anxiety can now be considered in the context of the condition of split consciousness. In summary so far, Owens's understanding of the traumatic nature of the English Reformation, and as it was evidenced on stage, may serve as a fitting backdrop for the original formation of the Cartesian Split complex. The myth of this complex has been interpreted as the splitting of consciousness, in which the original structure of consciousness has dissociated into multiple, quasi-conscious, and symmetrical fragments. In this case, the two most prominent fragments would be the Orthodox and the Protestant views regarding the Eucharist. Recall that split consciousness is given by two conflicting opinions about the same object.

For whatever reason, and for whatever merit, legitimate questions had now been raised concerning this most important ritual. Where once there was one certainty and one interpretation, there were now two very large doubts. Each side had very different opinions as to how the miracle could actually happen, who was authorized to perform it, and how the individual was to understand it.

From an outside perspective, both sides of this debate must be considered as equally conscious. Both sides still performed the ritual of communion, and both sides emphasized direct experience. However, each had two radically different opinions about this one event. Crucially, it seems that neither argument by itself was entirely convincing. Both had valid complaints about the other, and both accused the other of deceit, blasphemy, and idolatry. It is exactly as if two opposite hands were cut-off from each other, but living on, with each unable to affect the other. Thus, the right hand did not know what the other is doing, nor the left of the right. The anxiety of this tension is likely to have coincided with the fascination of seeing graphic displays of bodily dismemberment on stage.

Recall that my argument is that the Cartesian Split does not signify a split between consciousness and the unconscious. If it was formed, as a cultural complex, during the English Reformation, this aspect can also be observed in those original debates. That is, if the unconscious in the overall Christian myth is symbolized by the ultimate beyond, the realm of the hereafter, then it can be seen that neither side of the debate lost the integrity of this fundamental vision. Both Catholic and Protestant readily acknowledged the reality of the beyond and of the sacred. Rather, they differed fundamentally on the crucial question as to how this reality manifests in our world, and more importantly, how the individual may gain access to it. If anything, the heightened tension of the debate can only reveal an increased amount of attention toward the existence and modalities of the unconscious, but with two very different *conscious* attitudes toward it.

Parallels may also be drawn back to the mythic sources used for amplification of this condition. Recall that creation myths come in two general forms. The first are the mostly positive ones, in which a god is split up or dismembered, contributing to human culture. The second are the more negative ones, in which a human is dismembered by a god, which is harmful to culture. This can also be seen in the transformation of the saint play. The original saints were imitators of Christ, and through this identification, were able to bear the suffering of dismemberment, and this provided a cultural benefit. This is therefore a close analog to a positive myth of splitting. By contrast, Faustus is an anti-saint, and so his all-too-human failings make him unable to process what is happening to him, resulting in a bitter tragedy, being dismembered in the end by Mephistophilis. Also, the audiences were likely somewhat disturbed upon watching the final scene, and so this is an analog of a negative myth of splitting.

A specific parallel can also be made to the Gnostic myth, in terms of the resulting cultural divide. Recall that in this myth, humanity was seen to be divided between the Right and the Left, or those more psychical versus those more material, who each employed different ways of thinking. The Right was characterized more by abstract thought, whereas the Left more by concrete thought. In the case of the nature of the bread, the Protestants would then be the modern Right, seeing the bread as only a representation of Christ's flesh, with the actual miracle occurring only in the mind, through a statement of faith. The Catholics would be the Left, understanding the bread as being physically the same as Christ's body, and with the miracle being performed in the moment, in physical form. From the perspective of the Gnostic, neither the mind nor the body is adequate to express the ultimate truth, which is the realm of pure Spirit. It is for this reason that both sides are destined to be divided against each other, indefinitely, and this can also be seen in the unresolved tension between Catholics and Protestants. Interestingly, our modern political associations of party lines somewhat mirror this. The "Right" is generally understood to be more religious, with "Left" as more materialistic.

Thus, *Dr. Faustus* may indeed be a reliable historical record of an instance of split consciousness, revolving around the conflicting opinion on the nature of personal salvation. Two quasi-conscious opinions have formed where once there was one, and both have valid arguments, with neither one able to affect the other. At the cultural level, this can be seen in the long-standing conflict of opinion between two groups, within the same overall faith. As this is applied to the play itself, it can be seen in the fact that two very different interpretations can be made from the same play, along these two lines.

Faustus's internal split

Split consciousness is also characterized by internal contradiction, in which a single statement might be made which is internally incoherent. This is naturally best seen when it manifests at the individual or intrapsychic level. As Freud originally offered, the splitting of the ego is demonstrated by the simultaneous acknowledgment and disavowal of some single difficult reality. This very tendency is also uniquely expressed in the play, particularly from Faustus himself, and this is worth a detailed study.

In a sense, Faustus can be seen as an embodiment of all the anxieties and doubts that were occurring during the English Reformation. Not only can his single tragedy be understood by audiences in two different ways, but he himself understands his own singular situation in two different ways. This manifests in a terrific display of internal contradiction, as he wavers back and forth over his decision, agonizing over all the possible implications. However, he does this in a very paradoxical manner, full of irony. Rather than calmly weighing his alternatives, and being able to stand back from both of them, they seem to simultaneously occupy his statements and actions, manifesting in the kind of behavior Freud noted, where a contradiction is noted "in the same breath."

To introduce such themes, I rely on Kirschbaum (1977), who writes on exactly this aspect. Interestingly, he makes an overall observation that modern commentary on *Dr. Faustus* seems often to neglect the actual text (p. 87), not unlike current debates on Descartes. However, he specifically focuses on one aspect of the original text that has not received enough attention, which is especially relevant to my study. This is Marlowe's masterful use of "compressed dramatic irony" (p. 98), with which he shows Faustus's internal contradictions, his "disjunct character" (p. 96). Such a description can easily be imagined to be related to split consciousness. Also, Kirschbaum's notion that an irony is prevalent, and yet not well explored, is strikingly consistent with Freud's observation that the splitting of the ego is something both familiar and unusual at the same time.

At times, Faustus appears to deny any kind of life after death, either heaven or hell. He might consider these fanciful realms to be nothing but foolish superstition. With this understanding, he has nothing to fear by selling his soul, only gains to be made. However, after Mephistophilis assures him that hell is very real, and that Faustus is going there, Faustus mocks him for his cowardice and imagines himself to be all-powerful from his bargain (Kirschbaum, 1977, pp. 96–97). However, this is clearly ironic as it does not make any sense to revel in your divinely bestowed powers if the principles of the beyond are not really real. Further, there would be no need to boast if he was not truly afraid.

Similar behavior is noted regarding Faustus's belief in repentance from the God he denies. At times, he believes himself to be beyond all possibility of redemption; forgiveness may as well not even exist. However, at the same time, he is constantly reminded of that very possibility. Time and time again, he is offered a chance to repent, but he forcibly denies it. But it does not make any sense to have to constantly deny a God who does not exist, nor to constantly deny the possibility of repentance when those possibilities themselves keep manifesting. Thus Kirschbaum (1977) notes that Faustus "—characteristically—affirms the God whom he has just denied" (p. 99).

Such "compressed dramatic irony" shows up in many other forms, also in terms of how Faustus tried to relieve himself of the anxiety of his internal contradictions. His favored method is to indulge in various sensual comforts as if to convince himself that the present world is the only reality. Faustus desires the most beautiful wife because he is "wanton and lascivious." However, as he imagines how this will quell his fears, he simultaneously admits to himself that to do so will only make his final damnation all the more real (Kirschbaum, 1977, p. 100). Similarly, in another scene, he desires Helen of Troy, but his words are, as Kirschbaum states, "fraught with dramatic irony." Faustus himself acknowledges the epic danger of her beauty, that which caused the Trojan war, and also compares her to a succubus. But in the very same passage, he imagines that heaven itself could be found in her lips (p. 106).

Shortly before Faustus's death, his servant is "struck by the inconsistency of his master's character." Faustus had just written out his will, so he must have believed that the end was coming. But instead of acknowledging the dark implications of this, he frolics at supper, with "such belly-cheer" that has never been matched (Kirschbaum, 1977, p. 103). After agonizing with the decision for the entire play, this seems quite odd. And in the final scene, Faustus does indeed show his fears, so the cheerful supper is clearly a simultaneous acknowledgment and disavowal of his impending doom.

Kirschbaum (1977) suggests the most dramatic presentation of the "pervading irony" comes in the final moments, as Faustus goes over his wretched position one last time. Amazingly, he simultaneously presents himself as both a tragic failure and a legend in his own time. In the very same sentence, he laments how he has lost both Germany and the world, but also boasts of how much they will all eventually regard his accomplishments. Thus, his egotistic pride shows up in his very insistence of his damnation (p. 105).

The residual memory

Overall, on the basis of these symbolic resonances, the English Reformation is a likely backdrop for the formation of the Cartesian Split cultural complex. This is particularly well evidenced in the modes of theatrical presentations of human dismemberment, its core archetype, during this tumultuous period. It would be fair to say that this tumult has not yet been adequately resolved, if even recognized. Certainly, the exact terms of the original debate have not survived to the present day; there are no longer any heated debates on the substance of bread and wine, or the nature of immediate, personal salvation. Also, *Dr. Faustus* is no longer a popular performance. However, it can equally be argued that the original tension has not disappeared, but merely gone underground, and is now being expressed in new ways.

A penny for the Guy

One such potential new expression deserves special mention, and this is the curious legacy of Guy Fawkes. Fawkes was an Englishman who occupied a prominent role in the efforts of the Reformation and later became memorialized in unusual ways. This memory therefore serves as a very convenient bridge between the proposed original event and the present day. According to legend, Fawkes was the central figure of the infamous gunpowder plot, the failed attempt by Catholic loyalists to blow up the Protestant-leaning Parliament, in 1605. The coup was successfully put down, and Fawkes was captured and singled out as the leader. Convicted of high treason, he was tortured on the rack for days. In the end, he was, fittingly, dismembered. He was drawn and quartered, with his scattered remains sent across the kingdom to celebrate England's survival. Fawkes was perhaps our culture's first terrorist.

In commemoration of the victory against the terrorists, Parliament declared the fifth of November to be a recurring celebration. Church attendance was made mandatory, and effigies of Fawkes and other Catholic figures were to be burned in public, during what is now called Bonfire Night. Also, the cellars of Parliament were ceremoniously checked for explosives every year. These practices have continued up until the modern day. Selwood (2015) dryly notes that any foreign tourist, perhaps seeing such spectacles for the first time, would rightly observe that the country has "more than a hint of unresolved religious tension" (para. 3).

This practice is fraught with irony, in a way that is consistent with the themes presented above. Even without asking any questions, a foreign visitor would certainly find it strange that such violent and sensational spectacles would be needed to be re-enacted so dramatically every year. This applies particularly to the checking of cellars, where surely there are no actual expectations of finding actual explosives. But one wonders what kind of unconscious fears may still exist, that would perhaps be quelled by making sure there is no danger, more than 400 years later. It is as if the terrorists do still live on, only in the underground cellars of the mind, and such rituals are the only way to quell these uncomfortable doubts. Thus, by the mere presence of these rituals, they seem to simultaneously acknowledge and disavow a single difficult memory. It is also ironic that a day of freedom, associated with breaking with the orthodox rules of Rome, would be commemorated with mandatory church attendance. It is noted, however, that this mandate was later repealed.

However, perhaps the most interesting story is with the ritual figure of Guy Fawkes himself. The annual practice of burning him in effigy is itself a kind of theatrical performance that strongly resonates with Owens's (2005) understanding of the saint play. She notes that in the course of transformation from the originals to *Dr. Faustus*, there was also an intermediate point in which the exact same saint plays were being performed, only with the roles simply reversed. The torturer suddenly became the protagonist, as with the case of Henry VIII, and the suffering Catholic, the antagonist (pp. 44–46). Thus, the ritualistic burning of Guy Fawkes, which was done in the same fashion, may also be seen as a reflection of a need to keep some memory of this transformation alive.

However, the fact that this ritual is mostly celebrated and enjoyed indicates that Guy Fawkes may not be held to be entirely antagonistic. There are also some ironies noted in the way the effigies are built. At one time, it was evidently common for small children to build them, and to use them in tandem for asking for money, "a penny for the Guy." The dolls at this point are rather innocuous, almost endearing, and obviously are useful in invoking some kind of sympathy. This is a stunning irony, considering the eventual intended use of the doll. To draw a modern parallel, it would be equivalent to a child carrying a likeness of Osama bin Laden, and using it to ask for gifts. For one, parents would never let their child do such a thing, and if they did, the child would likely only get looks of disgust. In America, someone would likely be arrested and interrogated. In short, if Guy Fawkes was really regarded unequivocally as a terrorist, his dolls would not be prepared in such a manner. This can only betray the existence of some unconscious doubts, that perhaps he has been unfairly villainized, and his annual performance in a kind of modernized saint play may indeed be an unconscious reflection of this.

This kind of re-evaluation may have even swung all the way to the other extreme. Over the course of time, perhaps so slow that it was hard to notice, Guy Fawkes has become for many people today the exact opposite of a public enemy. Instead, most ironically, his iconic mask is a symbol of individual liberty against oppressive governments. This transformation is well captured in Alan Moore's seminal graphic novel, *V for Vendetta,* written in the late 1980s. Today, anti-establishment riots are heavily populated with Guy Fawkes masks. Overall, if Fawkes is a figurehead for the original religious debate, it seems as if an underlying tension has not been resolved at all. On the contrary, it seems to be strongly demanding a fresh look.

Religious dualism

There are likely a very wide variety of other modern cultural expressions that can be seen along these lines. The Reformation was undoubtedly a tumultuous period, which must have left a mark in all social spheres. However, I am primarily interested in how this mark shows up as the Cartesian Split complex, and in Anglophone academics, in which it has a unique expression. The image of a burning Guy Fawkes may be enigmatic to many, but only the philosophically minded academic is similarly occupied with the eternal "problem" of mind-body dualism, and to this I now return.

Earlier, I proposed that the Anglophone academic is but the voice of a larger Anglophone cultural complex. I then showed how the overall academic debate bears the marks of cultural fragmentation and unusual persistence. Now, after having just established a possible historical and cultural foundation, featuring the same patterns, I may now be able to establish a firmer link between the Anglophone academic and its larger culture, which is likely to have residual religious tension. This connection may seem strained, given the very different natures of the terms of the two debates, and the drastically more secular nature of the academic debate. And yet, that would exactly be the expected nature of an unconscious cultural complex. The modes of expression may change, but the overall pattern, and the specific feeling-tone, remains.

On the other hand, it may not be too daring at all to suggest that the ongoing academic debate is, in a sense, still quite religious. This can be seen in at least the overall pattern of behavior. In both cases, you have an elect minority of highly trained specialists, debating over the exact relationship between body and soul. There is also a "lay" audience, who is presumably interested in the results, and to which the elite feel a responsibility in educating. Also, although the salvation of the soul is no longer at stake, at least not explicitly, a requisite kind of devotion to the subject can easily be observed. This can be seen in the excessive amount of attention to detail to the philosophical subject. As Cottingham noted, some of our best minds have "devoted" an enormous amount of attention to the subject, regardless of how well they have understood Descartes.

Overall, from a broader perspective, the entire history of the debate on dualism can be compared to a community of elect theologians, performing a kind of biblical exegesis. Only in this case, the new scripture is an anonymously published book of Meditations, which, fittingly, concerns the nature of the soul, and also its relationship to God. These new theologians pore over every small detail in the original texts, correcting translations, and searching for the true meaning, exactly as a biblical scholar might. Whether or not they agree with what is stated is of secondary importance.

The typical student in Philosophy 101 is taught Cartesian dualism in detail, usually such that they may later refute it. This is because it is assumed to be dominant outside the halls of the elect, as a beguiling yet flawed solution to an important problem, fitting only for the naïve. What else could this be compared to besides a kind of religious training, with a structured pedagogy, designed to train new clergy on the proper interpretation of scripture, such that the lay population may be taught properly, and saved from the error of their ways?

The splitting of substance

It is also striking to note how close some of the terminology is, which might further validate the connection I am trying to make. It seems to me that the most pointed critiques of Cartesian dualism occur when it is expressed as a *substance* dualism, that is, as a firm distinction between two different *things*. Descartes did explicitly argue that mind and body are substances, and also that they are distinct, but he also argued for their "substantial union," as noted in earlier sections. And yet, the latter argument is frequently neglected, with the focus remaining only on the problematic distinction between two different substances. In short, it seems that the trigger word for the complex is *substance*.

When Descartes' philosophy is presented in these terms, it seems to generate unusually strong opinions. The response is generally some form of incredulity. Clearly, it is said, this is wholly wrong, for it is manifestly impossible for two different substances to interact. Even a simpleton can understand this, and it is indeed very odd that the father of modern philosophy could have ever duped himself into believing such absurdity.

However, it seems that such opinions are usually formed without ever taking the time to understand the meaning of the original terms, specifically *substance*. Descartes (1985) defines substance as "a thing which exists in such a way as to depend on no other thing for its existence" (p. 210). Strictly speaking, only God is a substance in this sense, but Descartes does recognize secondary substances, among God's creations. However, the crucial qualifier for this kind of substance is that its existence depends only on "the help of God's concurrence," whereas non-substances depend on other created things. For Descartes, mind and body are proper substances, belonging to this former category (p. 210). Clearly, Descartes uses this term in a drastically different manner than we do today, particularly given our more materialistic and secular biases. In my opinion, in its original usage, there seems to be nothing in the term that would necessarily dictate manners of mutual interaction. By contrast, for the modern critic of substance dualism, the very idea of "two different substances" seems to immediately lend itself to the conviction that it must be somewhat "radical," and therefore necessarily include all the well-documented problems of Cartesian Interactionism.

The question would then be, where does this conviction on the nature of *substantial* differences come from? If I am right about the relationship between this complex and the conflict of the English Reformation, one cannot help but look closely at the axis of the Reformers' agenda, the rejection of the ritual of the Eucharist. Specifically, I look closely at the rejection of transubstantiation, the miracle of transformation from common bread to Christ's flesh, or, in other words, *the transformation between two radically different substances*, one mundane, and the other divine. This was the miracle understood to be performed by the clergy, on behalf of God.

It must be significant that this doctrine was held to be unquestionably true, by most of the population, for centuries, both within and outside of England. Then, in a very short period of time, it was suddenly called into doubt, and replaced with two warring factions. Whereas one side outright rejected this doctrine, the other side reinforced it, with even larger conviction. Before the Reformation, there was perhaps no need to defend it so rigorously; it was a matter of accepted faith, and faith was a gift of Grace. Thus, both extremes can be seen to be reflective of a sudden and discomforting doubt concerning the exact relationship between mundane substance and divine substance. Or, in other terms, between bread and flesh, between the human body and Christ's body. Perhaps this doubt has now been extended and expressed in modern philosophical terms.

When the notion of substantial relationship is presented in the form of *res extensa* and *res cogitans*, there seems to be an immediate suspicion. As soon as the distinction is made in terms of substance, something deep inside of us seems to be incredulous. It is as if there is an unresolved doubt, right in the middle of this seemingly innocuous philosophical notion, concerning how the mundane is related to the divine. The myth of the Cartesian Split says that the two substances are radically and fundamentally separate. One cannot interact with the other, and by extension, nor can one transform into the other. Perhaps as a defense mechanism, instead of fully recognizing and internalizing this doubt, the overall distinction itself is wholly rejected. However, simply on the basis that the rejection has to be continually made, this might only reinforce the unfortunate fact that what it rejects exists. The Cartesian Split is both acknowledged and disavowed at the same time. In this way, it is not only symptomatic of split consciousness—it is itself split consciousness.

Substantial epochs

It is now possible to sketch out a possible timeline for the development and transmission of the Cartesian Split cultural complex over the centuries. The original container for this potent psychological dynamism appears to have been Dr. Faustus himself. Then, when the popularity of the stage play began to wane, it was perhaps transferred to the effigies and rituals of Guy Fawkes. Again, both figures were central to the religious fervor of the time, and both suffer violent and gruesome fates. Although, over time, there is a transformation in sentiment. The original audiences of Dr. Faustus, both Catholic and Protestant, likely enjoyed watching Faustus's tragic end. Guy Fawkes, on the other hand, began to take on some sympathetic overtones over time, indicating that he may not be all that bad. Perhaps it is around this time that the complex began to be interested in philosophy, looking for a new enemy.

It turns out that most of the sources of the Cartesian myth are restricted not just to Anglophone academics, but to *20th century* Anglophone academics. This has been noted already by others (Baker & Morris, 2002, p. x; Bolton, 1999; Cottingham, 1998, p. 2; Sorell, 2005, p. xx). Although misunderstandings and controversy concerning Descartes goes all the way back to his time, the content and tone of this current controversy seems to be uniquely different, and seems restricted to the 20th century. The earliest source I could find of the distinct Cartesian Split myth, in English, was Lovejoy's (1955) *Revolt Against Dualism*, originally published in 1928, and in this he references a 1926 news article (p. 2). Lovejoy's rhetoric indeed suggests that this was an original presentation, at least to him. This would make sense, as this shortly follows the time at which Descartes' work was first widely made available in English, with the Haldane and Ross translation, originally published in 1911 (Cottingham et al., 1985, p. viii).

Before this time, there may have been English commentary constitutive of this myth, but it is not prominent. On the contrary, for at least one prominent source, it is conspicuously missing. Writing before this time, Thomas Huxley (1892), in the prologue to his *Essays upon Some Controverted Questions*, approaches the subject in a very "un-Cartesian" way. He writes at length upon the subject of how the supernatural should now be understood against the newly introduced "natural" theory of Darwinian evolution. Remarkably, he frames this discussion with a classic Mirrored Worlds view. "Nature," in this case, is the "tangible, commonplace, orderly world," which is "surrounded and interpenetrated by another intangible and mysterious world," the world of "Supernature" (pp. 2–3). Such a "primitive dualism," according to Huxley, is thousands of years old, and instead of being a target of rejection, is only just then being re-evaluated (pp. 2–3). Huxley then delves into a wide range of heated disputes, fittingly, of a religious nature.

What is most remarkable is that for Huxley, Descartes is not the author of any kind of a problematic "dualism" between these two worlds. In fact, Huxley (1892) is concerned that it is *the religious debate* of his time that might result in a tragic split between them. Specifically, he is worried about this debate "cutting the Universe into two halves, one natural and one supernatural." What is even more remarkable about this account, is that Descartes' name is in fact invoked in this section, but in a positive light. Descartes' formulation, according to Huxley, actually leads to a position *where both worlds can co-exist*, only with a new criterion for truth in the supernatural world (pp. 26–27).

Thus, it is possible that the Anglophone complex, which was long concerned about the *substantial* differences between body and soul, human and divine, immediately found a new interest, in the early 20th century. This would have been the words of a long-dead French philosopher, offering intriguing meditations on the *substance* dualism between body and mind, which was only just then becoming more readily available in English. Huxley was likely reading Descartes in the original French or Latin.

Such a supposition of timing may have further empirical evidence, with the help of modern digital research. The internet search giant Google offers an impressive tool called Ngram, which can search for keywords across millions of scanned books, over time. Although surely there are some inaccuracies, I used this tool to see if any indication could be made on the timeline of popularity for these topics. I searched for the phrases "Guy Fawkes," "Cartesian dualism," and "Cartesian Split," all case-insensitive. The search period was from 1800 to the present, and of course in English, excluding fiction. I applied a moderate smoothing factor of 20, which is just an averaging function. The results are shown below.

This graph seems to support the timeline offered above. Notice how the popularity of Guy Fawkes begins to decline just as Cartesian dualism begins to rise, toward the end of 19th century. It is likely that these were based on personal translations of Descartes, or perhaps on problematic

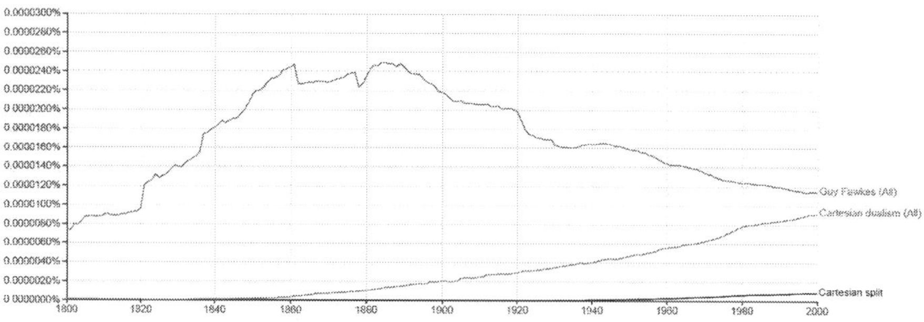

Figure 7.1 Ngram search results, by Michel et al.

early English translations that were extant around this time. This is because the definitive Haldane and Ross translation was published only a few decades later, in 1911. Perhaps this edition was a response to previously published translations, which were incomplete or flawed in comparison, or perhaps in response to Huxley's interest. In any case, shortly after this, in the early 1920s, as the Haldane and Ross edition was spreading, Guy Fawkes takes a sharp turn down, also around the time of Lovejoy's work in 1928. From this time forward, the two take on opposite trends. Another step change appears in the 1970s, with an increase of interest on dualism. Recall that this is when I observed the first academic philosophers noticing a problem with contemporary discussions on Descartes, prompting a new round of debate. Right around this time as well, the Cartesian Split starts to rise, roughly coincidental to Hillman and Capra's work, which had the best rhetoric. And now here we are today, with interest continuing to rise, on all subjects evidently. The question is then, what next?

References

Baker, G. P., & Morris, K. J. (2002). *Descartes' dualism*. London, UK: Routledge.

Bolton, R. (1999). Dualism and the philosophy of the soul. *Sacred Web*, *4*. Retrieved from: http://www.sacredweb.com/online_articles/sw4_bolton.html

Cottingham, J. (1998). Introduction. In J. Cottingham (Ed.), *Descartes* (pp. 1–27). Oxford, UK: Oxford University Press.

Cottingham, J., Stoothoff, R., & Murdoch, D. (1985). Introduction. In *The philosophical writings of Descartes* (Vol. 1, pp. viii–x). Cambridge, UK: Cambridge University Press.

Descartes, R. (1985). *The philosophical writings of Descartes* (Vol. 1; J. Cottingham, R. Stoothoff, & D. Murdoch, Trans.). Cambridge, UK: Cambridge University Press.

Duffy, E. (2005). *The stripping of the altars: Traditional religion in England; c. 1400 - c. 1580* (2nd ed.). New Haven, CT: Yale University Press.

Graffman, E. (2017). On Gregory Bateson's epistemology, his definition of mind, and its solution to the Cartesian dualism or mind-body problem. *Rocznik Naukowy Kujawsko-Pomorskiej Szkoły Wyższej w Bydgoszczy. Transdyscyplinarne Studia o Kulturze (i) Edukacji*, *12*, 146–157.

Hodge, K. M. (2008). Descartes mistake: How afterlife beliefs challenge the assumption that humans are intuitive Cartesian dualists. *Journal of Cognition and Culture*, *8*(3–4), 387–415.

Huxley, T. H. (1892). *Essays upon some controverted questions*. New York, NY: D. Appleton.

Johnson, G. (1997). Competing narratives: Retrieved February 26, 2017, from: http://gregscouch.homestead.com/files/henry8.html

Kirschbaum, L. (1977). Marlowe's Faustus: A reconsideration. In I. Ribner (Ed.), *Doctor Faustus: Text and major criticism* (pp. 87–106). Indianapolis, IN: Bobbs-Merrill.

Lovejoy, A. O. (1955). *The revolt against dualism: An inquiry concerning the existence of ideas*. Lasalle, IL: Open Court Publishing.

Owens, M. E. (2005). *Stages of dismemberment: The fragmented body in late medieval and early modern drama*. Newark, NJ: University of Delaware Press.

Richard, J. (2019, November 8). Gruesome ways people were executed in the time of Henry VIII. Retrieved November 8, 2019, from Ranker website: http://www.ranker.com/list/gruesome-executions-time-of-henry-viii/jeffrichard

Selwood, D. (2015, November 5). *Forget the Guy Fawkes propaganda—The English Reformation was a violent catastrophe*. Retrieved from: http://www.telegraph.co.uk/news/religion/11976813/Forget-the-Guy-Fawkes-propaganda-the-English-Reformation-was-a-violent-catastrophe.html

Sorell, T. (2005). *Descartes reinvented*. Cambridge, UK: Cambridge University Press.

Trevor-Roper, H. R. (1999). *The crisis of the seventeenth century: Religion, the Reformation, and social change*. Indianapolis, IN: Liberty Fund.

Weber, M. (1946). Science and Vocation. In H. Gerth & C. W. Mills (Eds.), *From Max Weber: Essays in sociology* (pp. 129–156). New York, NY: Oxford University Press.

Wilson, M. D. (1993). *Descartes*. London, UK: Routledge, Taylor & Francis.

Chapter 8

The alien text

In review, here is the overall story I have thus far constructed: The English Reformation left behind an unresolved tension concerning the nature of mundane and divine substances, possibly accompanied with concerns of personal salvation. This has left its mark in many ways in Anglophone culture, but shows up specifically in the academic portion today, manifesting as a cultural complex, through greatly distorted claims on substance dualism.

This analysis may give the impression that the complex is entirely a symptom of an unresolved historical trauma. In other words, that it was *caused* by something that happened in the past. However, such a view would only be consistent with a Freudian complex. As I have stated, Jung differentiated his theory of complexes from Freud by emphasizing their prospective functions over their causal backgrounds. The goal was to try to understand what the complex was doing in the present moment, and what it may be anticipating, in terms of future growth of the personality. From this point of view, a complex can be imagined as being prospective the whole time, perhaps even arranging events in the past, solely in order to enact a future change. Because of this, Jung did not discount the importance of causal factors. In general, he was content with how those aspects were treated by the Freudian tradition, which became increasingly interested in the dynamics of adolescence and parenting.

By contrast, Jung began to focus more on adults who were struggling with finding new ways to live their lives, going forward. This was in service to a process he referred to as individuation. The question now, however, is what to do with these difficult memories and unresolved doubts, starting today. There is some good news here, concerning this prospective function. According to Jung, every complex is Janus-faced: One side looks back to the past, while the other side looks to the future. In other words, the very same thing that is difficult to experience now simultaneously has everything within it necessary to resolve the conflict. Often, the complex points to relief in a most unexpected place. This forward-looking face will be the overall spirit of this chapter.

Certainly, some part of the prospective function of this complex suggests a better understanding of the original subject matter: The philosophy of Descartes. However, I must re-emphasize that the psychological history I have constructed goes back to England, and not to France, nor to any other country where Descartes lived and worked. In terms of a depth psychological analysis, and the bringing forward of unconscious contents, such a change of scenery is entirely appropriate. Also, thus far I have only needed to reference Descartes' actual philosophy as a negative example, in order to extract the Cartesian myth out of it.

As such, one may wonder what relevance, if any, the actual Descartes has toward my subject. Earlier I stated that the complex may have transferred from Guy Fawkes to the words on the page from a French philosopher, in the early 20th century. However, there are any number of *English* figures upon which such a myth could have been similarly constructed. All that would be necessary to trigger the transference would be any kind of argument for a mind-body distinction. Again, such a dualism is as old as Plato, and not exclusively owned by Descartes.

It would have perhaps been much closer to the mark, geographically and historically, if the myth was built up over one of the Cambridge Platonists. This was a group of influential 17th-century English philosophers whose writings could have formed such a foundation because they made similar arguments. Hutton (2013) describes this group as being "all dualists for whom mind is ontologically prior to matter, and for whom the truths of the mind are superior to sense-knowledge" (para. 2). This is similar enough to Descartes' position, at least close enough to trigger an irrational reaction. Similarly, one wonders why nobody recoiled in horror when reading Hamlet's soliloquy, specifically when he says that "to be" is to ponder shuffling off the "mortal coil" of the body. Nor do we ever vilify Yeats for lamenting the soul being tied down to the body, or in his words, "a dying animal." None of this happened, obviously, the myth was built up over Descartes instead. I have tried in this study to de-emphasize Descartes, but the complex, it seems, does not allow it. The question then is: Why? What is the purpose? Where is it leading?

One of the more consistent features of the Cartesian Split complex is the curious reluctance to actually read the source material. It seems to go beyond mere neglect, and resemble more of an active avoidance. Remarkably, this tendency has been noted in all disciplines, with Ryle in philosophy, to Capra in the history of science, and Hillman in depth psychology. The latter example is perhaps the most striking, given that Hillman himself stated that Descartes, his career arch-enemy, lives in the *Meditations*, and implores that the book is where the battle is, yet fails to actually read it. This stark lacuna of attention is thus also a yawning abyss of opportunity.

Therefore, one would have to suppose that one of the purposes of all of this is to actually read Descartes again. However, this would have to be done with a radically fresh perspective, one that is concerned with the present-day problems, along with the new version of history. It would also be beneficial to keep in mind all the exaggerations and distortions that are common to the complex, some of which are diametrically opposed to the actual texts. I hope that the preceding chapters have provided the necessary material toward such an effort.

With this approach, however, we should be wary of the temptation to want to discover the "real" Descartes, once the mythological distortions have been recognized. I believe this would be doing the present work a disservice, as there is already a voluminous amount of material on the historical Descartes, from those who are more qualified than me. Rather, I want the complex I have identified to remain present, as a unique impetus toward a new and different reading. In other words, the two halves of the Janus-face must be kept together, or else we risk yet another unfortunate split.

Applying this approach to the case with Ash might lead to a tense but productive reunion. Ash might be recommended to have a frank conversation with Rand, but this time with a new perspective, an awareness of the central importance of Ash's own story. But this does not mean that the actual Rand might not yet be of some help. Actually, the awareness of the distortions might lead to Ash feeling that Rand is finally able to be seen for the very first time. However, Ash must stay in the present. Rand's actual historical story might be interesting and helpful, but only to the extent that by recalling it, it supports the new story being told.

In this way, to use Sorell's designations, I am more interested in the canonical Descartes than the historical Descartes. That is, I believe the words on the pages have more to offer us today than the "real" historical figure, to the extent the latter is even possible to understand. It was, after all, the words on the page which seem to have triggered the transference in the early 20th century, not so much the 17th-century philosopher himself. And so, it is to these words I now turn. For these reasons, all subsequent references to Descartes generally refer to the canonical aspect only, rather than to the historical author.

A re-reading along these lines is sure to yield new insights. Baker and Morris (2002) rightly observe that a close reading of these texts reveals an utterly "alien" perspective to modern notions (p. 59). And so, it is now worth posing some questions to this literary alien, to see what kind of new insights may be found, especially concerning the new problem I have seemingly uncovered.

There are two levels that this approach may take, corresponding to the two layers of the unconscious. The deepest layer, the archetypal, has within it the archetype of dismemberment, which can manifest in split consciousness. This can happen, in theory, to all human cultures. Thus, some of this material could conceivably be of use to a cultural complex apart from our own, that perhaps was built up with different manifest content.

The remainder of the material will likely only be of interest to the Anglophone Cartesian Split cultural complex, which concerns a religious doubt concerning the substantial relationship between body and soul, or mundane and divine. This particular, distinct complex was built up on top of the larger, more universal archetype, as all complexes do. For this reason, the texts which address both levels are certainly to be of interest to the Anglophone complex.

Overall, this is a surely a multifaceted problem, and so it is worth a final review of all elements that I have introduced thus far. Therefore, in the following sections, I will both review the main points of my overall interpretation, followed by a possible response, from this alien text.

Descartes' disclaimer

The first overall point I raised in this work is, simply, that Descartes is still vastly misunderstood. Although this was noted to be already known by the experts, I decided to present this idea to a wider audience, by focusing on Descartes' sailor on a ship passage. The conventional narrative is that Descartes' mind-sailor is a ghost, above and beyond the ship of the body, completely disconnected from it. The passage itself, however, outright contradicts this. Not only is Descartes' mind on the ship, constantly interacting with it, but beyond this, *the mind is the ship*. It is distinct, but it experiences reality as the ship does. If the ship runs onto a rocky shore, the mind feels the pain (Descartes, 1984, p. 56). This drastic disparity of meaning is consistent with the nature of unconscious complexes, as I have stated. The overall effect was to present the canonical Descartes as the best refutation against the modern "Cartesian" construction.

It is worth noting that such deliberate usage of irony is not new, as Baker and Morris, and also Cottingham, have previously employed it. It is simple and effective, and facilitated by the fact that most critiques come along with the unfortunate habit of taking Descartes' quotes highly out of context, or worse, not reading him at all.

It is common to not read Descartes because everyone already "knows" him. Recall that Ryle did not provide any direct quotes, nor any footnotes, and I found similar behavior in Capra and Hillman. Sheldrake provided a citation that did not check out, and evidently the editor did not feel the need to check this. And so, it is relatively easy to present the canonical Descartes as a counterargument to Descartes. However, the most interesting aspect of this is how Descartes (1984) himself seems to have anticipated exactly such behavior. In the preface to the *Meditations*, he writes:

> I do not expect any popular approval, or indeed any wide audience. On the contrary I would not urge anyone to read this book except those who are able to meditate seriously with me, and to withdraw

> their minds from the senses and from all preconceived opinions. Such readers, as I well know, are few and far between. Those who do not bother to grasp the proper order of my arguments and the connection between them, but merely try to carp at individual sentences, as is the fashion, will not get much benefit from reading this book.
>
> (p. 8)

Remarkably, in a single paragraph, Descartes manages to effectively dismiss most critical commentary in the subsequent 400 years. What is more, he seems to have uncannily predicted their behavior, as seen in Ryle, Capra, and Hillman. Also, it is worth noting that Descartes' recommended approach to his writings could even be called a holistic approach, in that it is stated that you must read the whole work, in order to properly understand it, or indeed any part of it. This contrasts with a reductionist or atomistic approach that focuses on an understanding of parts in isolation, to build an understanding of the whole. Recall that this latter approach to understanding is essentially how Capra defines the "Cartesian" mechanistic approach, and so again, the canonical Descartes is an uncannily effective counter to this.

Another interesting aspect to this prefacing statement is that Descartes is just as distrustful of preconceived opinions as he is of the senses. Almost universally, however, it is specifically the doubting of the senses and the body that constitutes his dubious legacy. The doubting of preconceived opinions in the mind, by contrast, seems to be a widely accepted virtue, but this aspect is commonly neglected. This is all the more important to reconsider because it is now exactly the preconceived opinions of Descartes himself that should be now doubted.

The evil genius

As has been covered, there is a vast amount of misunderstanding concerning Descartes' philosophy, and even how to approach it, but perhaps the most striking distortion is that of Descartes himself. Specifically, I am referring to the larger-than-life status he assumes when his ongoing legacy is discussed. In my review, this came out most prominently in Capra, who envisioned the entire history of modern science as the unfolding of a single, nefarious Cartesian agenda. This influence was so powerful that even Einstein could not break free. This figure I termed the Evil Genius, and the theme is also related to the endless supply of Heroic Transcenders, which all tragically fail in the end. It is as if Descartes has become an all-powerful, immortal spirit, who is able to control our thoughts against our better judgment, requiring continual challenges to his persistent influence.

It is redundant at this point to show how this is a mythic distortion, far removed from the actual texts. And yet, it turns out that such a villainous figure does make a significant appearance in the *Meditations*. However, in a stunning irony, it is Descartes who is the unfortunate victim of this influence. This is the work of the demon deceiver, who has the power over Descartes' thoughts, and devotes all of his energies to force untrue beliefs onto him. A significant portion of the book is dedicated toward exorcising this highly pernicious influence. If it were in fact true that a Cartesian Evil Genius was presently in control of us today, it would be highly worthwhile to see how Descartes himself managed to get free of the demon, that which was later named after him.

This specific irony has been noted by at least two other commentators. Baker and Morris (2002) hint at it in a footnote (p. 2), and Bracken (2002) captures it with a powerful closing statement in his book on Descartes (p. 131). However, neither was able to fully develop this irony from the standpoint of psychological complexes. From this perspective, it is not so much an irony as it is the normal course of events. If a complex is given full range of expression, it can often turn everything upside-down, and sometimes force the very opposite of the consciously chosen direction. Jung sometimes referred to this behavior as an *enantiodromia*. This is a process by which a complex can serve as a renewal of the personality, by forcing a confrontation with the shadow, or what was once rejected. This might manifest, as an example, with someone obsessing over an enemy so much that they become the very thing they once despised. In this aspect, complexes have an undoubtable trickster nature to them.

It is then more than fitting that Jung (1934/1969) refers to this aspect of complexes as "impish tricks," played on us by complexes, behaving like "Descartes' devils" (p. 97), forcing us to do exactly what we do not wish. Jung is almost certainly referring to the demon deceiver here, but curiously, he makes it plural. This is perhaps due to the fact that in that very paragraph, he was also referring to the tendency of the psyche to split into multiple fragments, each with a noted degree of consciousness.

And so, there is an extraordinary confluence of potential meanings grouped around Descartes' demon. First, Descartes has become the very same demon he once tried to exorcise. Notably, this attempt was unsuccessful, in a very ironic fashion. Second, this irony seems to be imploring us to find a solution in the middle of the problem, as complexes normally do. Third, in describing the problem of split-off complexes, Jung refers to one of Descartes' most novel contributions, the demon, but in an offhand way, that suggests that the exorcism of the demon might also be a solution to split consciousness. I will develop this notion further in later sections.

Cogito and consciousness

One of the first conclusions I made was that the Cartesian Split myth had an uncanny resemblance to a creation myth, specifically one concerning the creation of consciousness. I also noted that Descartes, the human being, could not possibly have been involved in any part of this, as human consciousness in some form has existed since at least the first written records. However, Descartes certainly belongs in the history of the *word* consciousness, or what might be termed the consciousness of consciousness.

However, this may not proceed in the way commonly accepted. As Baker and Morris (2002) note, it is common to assume that the first appearance of this word follows from Descartes, particularly from his usage of the Latin *conscientia*. Historically, this term had a varied and complicated range of meanings, but most were centered on a sense of morality, which relates it to our word conscience (p. 102). However, according to many, Descartes "innovated" the modern usage of the term *consciousness* by liberating it from *conscientia*, and therefore away from the old notions of morality. In this way, it is assumed that Descartes essentially replaced this notion with *cogitatio*. However, Baker and Morris note that this interpretation is heavily contaminated with the Legend, and is not well supported by the evidence. In fact, under scrutiny, Descartes does not use the term heavily, and where he does, he frequently maintains the original usage (p. 101). Also, it is noted that the overall moral dimension of Descartes' philosophy is usually neglected by Anglo-American interpreters (p. 124). Overall, it seems that conventional notions of consciousness cannot be so easily be assigned to Descartes' *conscientia*.

However, in any case, the subject material of the *Meditations* certainly touches upon aspects of whatever we now call consciousness. Perhaps the real challenge is in more precisely defining the term, and locating it for future use. In one interpretation, Descartes' *conscientia* bears a noteworthy resemblance to the definition of consciousness *as it is used in depth psychology*, both in its meaning, and its relationship to morality.

Morris (2017) interprets Descartes' *conscientia* in a way that is compatible with this view. Contrary to common interpretations, this version is not equivalent to common thinking, or even a higher-order version of it, which would amount to a "thinking of thinking." This would lead to an infinite regress, something Descartes noted and tried to avoid (pp. 13–14). Rather, Descartes could be arguing that *conscientia* is a certain aspect of thinking, something that is normally present, but *not normally recognized*. The task of the philosopher, with the help of the *Meditations*, might be to become gradually aware of this important aspect of thinking, through the process of reflection (p. 15). Morris then speculates that such reflection may also serve as the basis for better knowledge of one's moral character (pp. 19–20).

This interpretation can be positively compared to the term *consciousness* in Jungian psychology. For Jung as well, the faculty of consciousness is not the same as rote thinking. In his typology of personality, "thinking" is just one of four basic psychological functions, which may or may not be conscious. By contrast, consciousness is more fundamental, common to all functions, but is not always dominant. This also has moral implications. To illustrate this, consciousness can be imagined as a small island, surrounded by the dangers of the sea of the unconscious. Given that the unconscious is understood as essentially amoral, most failings of morality are due to a failure of consciousness, or in other words, a flood.

The *Meditations* offer a comparable view, in that the soul is surrounded by a vast number of doubtful objects, including not just the images from our senses, but also intellectual propositions. According to Baker and Morris (2002), the moral dimension of *cogitatio* involves the proper use of *judgment* regarding the truthfulness of all these propositions (p. 117). In the language of depth psychology, the island of consciousness must always be at least one degree removed from the turbid sea of unconsciousness, in order to maintain some degree of volition, and therefore a sense of moral responsibility. Jung (1958/1970) also describes consciousness in this way and notes its close ties with conscience and morality. Similarly, for Freud, conscience is built up over time from the ego's resistance to the amoral demands of the unconscious Id. Although, conscience does end up in the superego, which may only be partially conscious.

Baker and Morris (2002) also note that the word *consciousness* is extraordinarily difficult to define, and may in fact have a different meaning for every person (p. 124). This point seems to be well reflected in modern consciousness studies, which draws from many disciplines. For many researchers in neuroscience, consciousness is an illusion, a false reality superimposed upon the more primary hard-wiring of the brain. For those more inclined to consult the wisdom traditions, such as Buddhism, consciousness is the all-pervading stuff of the entire universe. So, either consciousness is nothing or everything. Or, perhaps both are right, and the term is just that slippery. For these reasons, I have used the language of myth as much as possible to describe the dynamics of consciousness. Descartes' approach might be comparable, given that it seems to emerge only after a prolonged battle with a demon, which is a figure from myth. Overall, it is enough for now to state that Descartes' notion of consciousness, in all its restrictive, moral, and dramatic senses, is worth a close consideration in this new field of study.

Depth psychology obviously makes usage of this term, in different ways, but perhaps also struggles with problems of defining it. This could be a real hindrance because, in this field, only consciousness can investigate the depths of the unconscious, and if the former is not adequately understood, the entire pursuit may be compromised. I have noted how various depth-oriented psychologists tend to conflate consciousness with the mundane "outer," and how this may create difficulty. Overall, it is useful to note that Descartes' attempts to define it are certainly no worse than modern attempts, and even if his definitions are not currently relevant, a close study of these first attempts might force current practitioners to develop better definitions.

In addition to the history of consciousness, Descartes also deserves more consideration in the history of the unconscious. As Eshleman (2007) states in "The Cartesian Unconscious," there is a basic, if rudimentary, model of unconscious influences in Descartes' work. Specifically, this is in his letter to Chanut, in which he describes his early fascination with the cross-eyed girl. Essentially, a memory was acquired by some strong experience with the girl in his childhood, and persisted until adulthood, until Descartes brought the memory fully to consciousness, at which time its influence was lessened. Eshleman argues from this that most commentators unfairly begin psychodynamic history with Leibniz, when it should, from this example, begin with Descartes (p. 169).

In my reading of Descartes, there are several other rudimentary forms of a psychology of the unconscious. First, there is the persistence of preconceived opinions, which take over his mind against his wishes (Descartes, 1984, p. 15), or in other words, unconsciously. Also, again, this comes in the form of a mythic personification, the demon deceiver, and this is commonly understood as a preferred expression of unconscious influences. Further, as Descartes tries to develop a method for addressing these influences, there are brief hints of the first stages of the Jungian method of active imagination (p. 17).

In summary, although Descartes did not create consciousness, he certainly attempted to define it. He also appears to be working with the dynamics between it and unconscious influences, in a way remarkably prescient to future psychologies. A careful review of these efforts might be constructive for similar efforts today, both in consciousness studies, and in the field of depth psychology.

Meditations on split consciousness

However, the dominant aspect of this complex is likely more concerned with the present nature of consciousness than with its definitions. In review, the symbolic imagery in the underlying myth suggests that consciousness itself has become split up. Something in the overall psyche has become fragmented, but the lines of fragmentation are not between consciousness and any object, or between consciousness and the unconscious, but within consciousness itself. This is given by a multitude of quasi-conscious fragments, with equivalent amounts of certainty. An image for this is a tragic dismemberment: The right hand has been cut off from the left, just as the left has from the right, and neither knows what the other is doing, and this condition is doggedly persistent.

At the archetypal level, this was seen in the Gnostic myth as the divide that ran through the whole of society. This divide was between the Right and the Left, or Psychics and Materials, and this correlated to the split between soul and body, heaven and earth. Each group was characterized by a certain way of thinking, one more representational and the other more literal. However, from the point of view of the Gnostics, or those on behalf of Spirit, they are all equally right and equally wrong. Their opinions and theories were all judged to be inarticulate and confused, due to unconscious influence from the rulers, the archons, who benefited from the division by maintaining control. Jung, in his attempts to describe a similar condition in modern times, painted a picture of a hopeless conflict between science and religion, East and West, and faith versus knowledge. Thus, at any level, anyone needing liberation from these deep divides has a real epistemological crisis on their hands.

As suggested previously, Descartes' work may uniquely concern this subject, particularly the *Meditations*. The opening paragraphs from the 1st Meditation features such a crisis, commensurate to the situations described above. And yet, these paragraphs have been read so many times by dedicated scholars, or not at all by others, that perhaps it is easy to underappreciate the severity of this crisis.

For whatever reason, Descartes (1984) finds himself in a highly dramatic situation, one which requires doubting everything he has ever learned, including everything taught in school, and everything else that was subsequently built on top of those first lessons. The entire edifice must be destroyed, a new foundation must be laid, and truth to be rebuilt from the ground up, in order to have any reliable knowledge. The task is an enormous one and must be done alone. The difficulty of such an undertaking is such that it should only be attempted once in one's lifetime (p. 12). It should go without saying that with such a comprehensive rejection, both sides of many arguments are all considered equally. In other words, the scope of material corresponds well to the constituents of split consciousness.

In addition to such high drama, this text is remarkable for one other reason. This is the oddly personal nature of the subject of the text. Descartes invites the reader to "meditate with me" in the preface, and he makes good on this invitation. In the very first paragraph, the reader is right there with Descartes, as he is meditating alone by a fire, with almost every argument made by an "I." It is easy to imagine you are in the very stove-heated room in which he supposedly made his philosophical discovery. Of course, this literary style is the very opposite of the caricature of the cold, detached, "Cartesian" scientist, one who strives to maintain a critical, objective distance from their products of the work, stripping all "I"s from their work.

And yet, Frankfurt (2008) notes that the "I" of the Meditations, is at the same time *not* the historical Descartes. In addition to the author at the time of writing, Descartes appears to also include within this "I" both prior versions of himself, as well as a version of himself as a general, human thinker. For this reason, the subject of the Meditations is sometimes called "the thinker." This invites any reader whatsoever, from any time, place, gender, or race, to meditate along with him, perhaps even from within the same "I." Perhaps this is not ultimately possible, but Descartes' attempt is at least intriguing and appropriate to his own philosophy (pp. 3–6). Further, it is highly appropriate for my study, if it truly addresses an archetypal situation, in the present, as I am suggesting.

Internalizing doubt

As stated in the preface, the thinker is concerned that only a few people are going to be able to meditate with him seriously, given the weight of the situation. It is far too easy for us today to say that we are going to be open-minded, that we are ready to turn a new leaf or to free our minds. However, I believe that these are mere utterances that do not weigh up to the depth of the concerns in the *Meditations*. Perhaps the best way to gauge whether the reader is "serious" enough, is to view it in terms of the archetype of dismemberment. As has been suggested, the images of dismemberment are uniquely powerful, because they remind us of our deepest fragility. This would be a fragmented consciousness, in which *nothing at all can be held to be true*. It is with this kind of crisis that the thinker is deeply troubled.

Fittingly, as Bordo (1987) has pointed out, what follows the preface is a real existential crisis, a level of doubt that invites a certain kind of madness. It is "a nightmare landscape," that is "invasive, vertiginous" (p. 14), and in which the subject experiences "hyperbolic doubt" (p. 120). This kind of drama is that which is sometimes missed, or at least not adequately appreciated (pp. 14–18). The thinker doubts his most secure and cherished beliefs. He doubts whether he is truly awake, or just dreaming, and even doubts the existence of God. The loss of God is not dramatic enough, however, because he inserts in God's place the demon deceiver, who is employing all his energies to deceive. From this pernicious influence, nothing can be said to be wholly certain, or at least not as initially perceived. This includes the possibility of perceiving that two plus three equals something other than five (Descartes, 1984, p. 25). This is a truly remarkable position of doubt for a famed mathematician.

The thinker has thus internalized a position of radical doubt, one that is commensurate to the tragedy of dismemberment. In other words, he has allowed the dire suspicion that the entirety of culture is hopelessly fragmented, with all of the experts at least partially wrong. The key move, however, is that the thinker brings it all inside, rather than simply bemoaning all those "others" for being hopelessly confused, allowing himself to avoid any personal responsibility. This is indicated in the overall structure of the entire essay, which almost resembles a dialogue, featuring an interminable back-and-forth of every kind of opinion. The thinker is arguing with himself and is relentless. Frequently, there is a paragraph that works out an entire proposition, point by point, only to be wholly rejected in the next.

This process is reflective of an anxiety of falling apart, but also of not even having parts. That is, there is the doubt of not having a body. This is, of course, one of the more notorious aspects of Descartes' arguments. However, I do not believe it suffices to say that he rejects his body simply because he is a rationalist. Rather, this particular notion may have been chosen, among many others, as a specific rhetorical device that is most effective toward conveying a specific kind of anxiety. If the text is followed closely, what could be more terrifying than to look at your own hand and suddenly suspect that it is not truly yours? Or worse, that it is a malicious deception, a false image forced upon you by a powerful Evil Genius, who is actively trying to deceive you? Perhaps there is no more powerful image of dismemberment than this.

The process of doubt

With an emphasis on such hyperbolic doubt, these Meditations certainly appear to be of a different kind of text. Morris (in press, 2017) argues that the text is unique because it implores the reader to do some additional philosophical work on their own. I am now suggesting that it implores additional psychological work. Working though complexes is a messy affair, and this complex would certainly be no different.

Hyperbolic doubt is more than just a position to be held, it is a *process*. This is a process by which all propositions and all preconceived opinions, even those that seem most certain, can be properly doubted. It might even be appropriate to say that the text accomplishes its goal if the reader begins to doubt that they are even holding the book. Overall, for these reasons, you cannot take any single line out of this work and use it to define what "Descartes" thinks. Again, the author explicitly warns against this. But, regrettably, this is what is usually done. It is easy to point to one section of the *Meditations,* such as the thinker doubting his body, and use that to condemn the thinker for lack of embodiment, rejection of the feminine, separation from nature, or any other position that one wishes to critique. However, if the entire proceeding is followed, the resulting doubt is powerful enough to doubt even those noble pursuits. This is not to say that they are ultimately wrong but that the pursuit may be more effective *if a certain state of mind is first established*.

In other words, the *Meditations* may be understood as a kind of litany, or as a psychological recipe, that aims to "cook up" a certain state of consciousness. In other words, it is *psychoactive*. Such an evaluation is harmonious with Lee (2013, pp. 6–13) and Bracken (2002, p. 29). Perhaps, if read in a certain way, it can do this every time it is read, like a magical spell, rather than serve as a dry historical record of a certain set of arguments. This is supported by the fact that toward the end of the *Meditations*, the thinker sets out to prove the very things he first doubted, as if he knows he now has a better mental apparatus with which to think about them. He proves that God exists, that truth can be reliably obtained, and again, that the soul is substantially united with the body. And so, the doubt is clearly a process, rather than an end in itself. Descartes (1984) says almost exactly this in the synopsis: "The great benefit of these arguments is not, in my view, that they prove what they establish." Rather, "the point is that *in considering these arguments we come to realize* [italics added]..." (p. 11). What is subsequently realized is that the soul has everything it needs within itself to know and understand truth. However, it is evidently latent and must be uncovered through some kind of process. Again, for this to occur, the author recommends that the text be read holistically, in the proper order, and not as a series of atomistic, disconnected arguments.

What is more, and perhaps puzzling, is that the thinker here seems to belittle his own prior position of radical doubt. Recall that he only wants a reader who is able to "meditate seriously with me," which includes doubting the reality of the world, and of the body. But at the end of the synopsis, he curiously states that "no sane person has ever seriously doubted these things" (Descartes, 1984, p. 11). This can be read in two different ways. Either Descartes is blatantly contradicting himself, or perhaps there is something else. He could be saying, as he said before, that this is a process you only have to go through once in your life. That is, the serious doubt is necessary only temporarily, in order to produce a certain moment of clarity, and afterwards, the old familiar notions of reality may be safely restored, in the same form as before. The difference is simply a new "knower." However, perhaps there is yet another way to read it. It could be taken to mean that "no sane person" can ever reach the necessary state of mind. In other words, in order to meet the real crisis properly, perhaps a temporary bout of insanity is not just an unfortunate precursor, but *may in fact may be required in order to produce the required solution.* Naturally, this is very far removed from how the text is usually read.

In summary so far, the *Meditations* can be read as a response to the archetypal condition of split consciousness. However, because of the unique nature of the phenomenon, a different psychological state is first required, and this could be the reason for the unusual structure of the text. This may be to induce in the reader a psychological process of radical doubt, instead of simply presenting an argument of doubt. In other words, it may be less a set of philosophical propositions, to be either validated or rejected, but more of an invitation to a psychological journey, to be either accepted or not.

For other reasons, at this point in the process, rational analysis alone is not likely to help the deeper psychological condition presently being addressed. Such a condition is already given by excessive fragmentation, not only within the whole psyche but within the very structure that apprehends. More ratiocination, that is, proposition "A" being favored over "B," and rejecting "B," would not be conducive to finding a solution, because it may be impossible to know if these are really two discrete propositions, or perhaps instead another reflection of the subject's own internal dissociation.

A singular truth

With conscious fragments everywhere, something singular appears to be required. In the 2nd Meditation, the thinker hints at this need, seeking a single, Archimedean point, upon which anything can be moved. Success may be found "if I manage to find just one thing, however slight, that is certain and unshakeable" (Descartes, 1984, p. 16). The thinker's only recourse is to focus rigorously on this "I" that is doubting everything, including the "I" itself. Can it be said that "I do not exist?" The thinker then has a singular insight. The answer to this last question is a resolute "No," for such a statement requires a thinker to think it. "This proposition, *I am, I exist,* is necessarily true whenever it is put forward by me or conceived in my mind" (p. 17). "I" is self-validating.

However, all those quasi-certain propositions are still surrounding the newly fortified "I." More work is required. In the 4th Meditation, the role of free will is explored. The thinker then realizes that he has the ability to withhold assent from all possible propositions. The thinker realizes that by withholding judgment, he is naturally exercising some innate faculty of judgment. In other words, he may be continually deceived by many dubious propositions, but at least he can always control the process of judgment (Descartes, 1984, pp. 39–43). Similar to the self-validating "I," the very act of doubting is something that cannot possibly be false, for to doubt the faculty of doubting is to in fact prove that it exists, *and* that it is necessarily reliable. Thus, in a single moment, a reliable foundation of knowledge has been finally found, as well as a form of undeniable existence. *Cogito, ergo sum.*

Naturally, this moment has been interpreted thousands of times, in many different ways, and my interpretation above fits in with this history. For this, I am following the best I have found from the dedicated scholars in philosophy. To these, I am emphasizing the psychoactive aspects of the text, as noted by Bordo and Lee. What I am now additionally contributing is another, more psychological interpretation. I believe this specific moment of an especially difficult meditation can also be expressed as a critical step forward toward a solution to split consciousness.

I will justify this claim further in the following sections. For now, two points will suffice. One, most basically, is that the text explicitly describes a process of bringing together conscious fragments. What started out as a myriad of divisions outside, became a myriad of divisions inside. This was carried out to the point of the highest possible position of doubt, in which no one fragment can be said to be true. Then, at some point, a single fragment is found to hold up as wholly true, even under this most radical doubt. Thus, a singular foundation may have been found, upon which subsequent knowledge can be built. Second, it is interesting to note the nature of one of the statements evaluated during this process. Bordo (1987) notes that the statement "I do not exist" amounts to what Descartes calls a "manifest contradiction," and this is echoed by another theorist as a "self-defeating" statement (p. 26). A statement described as such could also be compared to the internal contradictions common to split consciousness, as in a single statement consisting of two different positions. Therefore, this overall process would seem appropriate to such a condition.

A single sapling

Although the text thus far follows the work of a single thinker, it can also be seen to have a rather wide scope. That is, a singular foundation of knowledge may translate equally well to a large community of thinkers. It is clear that Descartes had this in mind, particularly in his preface to his *Principles of Philosophy*. In this text, Descartes (1985) boldly imagines the entirety of human knowledge as a single tree, with the root as metaphysics, the trunk as physics, and the branches as everything else (p. 186). His preferred metaphysics for this tree naturally follows from similar premises as covered in the *Meditations*.

Such an image might have been controversial in the 17th century, but would likely be forcefully rejected today. This would not be due to the fact that metaphysics, or even the version of it today which we now call philosophy, is now much less popular. Rather, it would be rejected on the basis of any discipline whatsoever being chosen as fundamental to all the others. Today, we live in an academic culture of extreme egalitarianism, where no one discipline may proclaim privileged access to fundamental truths, as pointed out by Rorty. There are of course many virtues to this. But might such a radical decentralization might also be vulnerable to a pathology of collective split consciousness? That is, if there are truly no "first principles," on what basis exactly should two scholars from different traditions converse productively on a single subject?

Recall that Kelso (2015) defined the Cartesian Split as "that fateful division that now dominates all *branches* of knowledge" [italics added] (para. 2). For better or worse, the tree has been broken. Perhaps Descartes has split his very own tree. It is beyond the scope of this work to argue whether or not such a tree may be regrown, or if first principles truly exist, and how they might form a common foundation. However, it is undeniable that we live in a time of heavy academic specialization, perhaps even fragmentation. There are more and more journals from every possible discipline and seemingly less and less collaboration. In such a climate, perhaps it is enough to at least meditate on the possibility of a single, foundational discipline.

Inoculation

The thinker now begins to focus more on the act of judgment, to see how this singular moment of truth might be extended any further. Descartes, in the 4th Meditation, explores more deeply the role of the will, in terms of making judgments. In one section, the doubt on having a body is revisited, this time with more detail, and from this new perspective.

Recall that split consciousness is characterized by entertaining multiple propositions about a singular reality, and each proposition has an equal amount of certitude. This situation is mirrored quite well by the thinker in this section. Descartes (1984) focuses on the idea of his body or his "corporeal nature." This time, however, he entertains two possible judgments on this (single) idea. Either the "I," the thinking thing, is distinct from the body, or is identical with it. Both are allowed to have equal claims of certitude (p. 41). Of course, it is only the former judgment that is claimed to be "Cartesian," but the canonical Descartes, at this point, refuses to decide. Crucially, a proper Cartesian doubt means not just doubting the body, *but doubting Cartesian dualism just as much.* Notably, the former proposition is eventually decided on, in the form of a substantial union, but this is the result of a process, not necessarily a self-contained truth.

This process is related to the usage of the will. Descartes (1984) makes the striking statement that, unless certain conditions are first met with regard to the exercise of will, simply the act of making a decision can be considered an error, regardless of whether the eventual choice ends up being true. This would be the case if the will happened to be extended beyond the reach of possible intelligibility. Thus, it is only with the proper exercise of the will, that absolute truth is guaranteed, regardless of the answer (p. 41). This is related to the critical moral dimension of the *Meditations.*

More importantly, Descartes (1984) subsequently states that the will is, in its essence, singular. It consists "simply of one thing which is, as it were, *indivisible*, it seems that its nature rules out the possibility of anything being taken away from it" [italics added] (p. 42). Again, this is a foundational realization, a singular solace, in the midst of a fragmented consciousness. The thinker seems to accept the possibility that both propositions are at least partially true, that he is both identical to the body and also distinct from it. However, crucially, he realizes in this moment that his thinking, or his judgment, need not necessarily be split up along these lines. In the free exercise of free will, he has the ability to temporarily withhold assent from either alternative. The thinker has thus found something inherently indivisible, or, in other words, *something that cannot possibly be dismembered.*

In this one important aspect, the will shares in the nature of the soul, which is also indivisible. In the 6th Meditation, Descartes (1984) recapitulates the special distinction of the soul, or mind, which for Descartes is an interchangeable term. First, "the mind is utterly *indivisible*" [italics added]. As summarized above, for all of the impressive displays of doubt, the thinker finds that it is impossible to divide the act of doubting into two, and this is also the case with thinking, as defined above. The soul is therefore immune *in essence* to the threat of dismemberment. This is not the case for the body, or even the idea of body, which is inherently divisible, and therefore prone to dismemberment. He even uses dismemberment explicitly as an example. "If a foot or arm or any other part of the body is cut off, nothing has thereby been taken away from the mind" (p. 59). This is therefore a statement of inoculation against the threat of tragic dismemberment by the demon deceiver. It is also worth noting that the notion of indivisibility can be related to Jung's individuation. This is a term he would often expand upon as "in-dividual," because it represents a condition of becoming an "indivisible unity" (Jung, 1954/1969, p. 275).

The theme of dismemberment also appears explicitly in other sections, in a similar manner. Descartes (1984) considers the situation of an amputee who still feels pain in the area of their missing limb. For this reason, among others, the thinker has reason to doubt the senses, and in how they report the state of the body (p. 53). Thus, in the inherent divisibility of matter, there is ample room for the demon to employ his tricks of deception. The only refuge is in the indivisible, singular moment of immediate awareness.

However, as demonstrated in the 4th Meditation, the crux of the moral problem lies in the proper use of judgment, which is in the soul. Therefore, for the thinker, it seems the body, and by extension all of matter, *is not inherently distrustful*. Rather, it seems that is only inherently divisible. The problem only arises when this aspect of matter is combined with a soul that has not yet mastered its usage of indivisible will. In such a case, the unrestrained will may lose its bearings, or become lost, in the divisibility of matter. It is perhaps from this combination, that the possibility of error emerges, in the form of flawed judgments concerning matter. Therefore, there is good reason to believe that, from this perspective, the thinker is actually more distrustful of the mind than the body. This is of course the opposite of the common caricature. As if to encapsulate this point, in the 2nd Meditation, the thinker states, "I am amazed at how weak and prone to error my mind is" (Descartes, 1984, p. 21).

Correspondingly, Descartes (1984) pays his respect to the body and its senses. He reasons that the senses perform their functions as best they possibly can, and thankfully, they "report the truth much more frequently than not" (p. 61). However, *it is up to the soul to make proper judgments,* about what the senses are reporting. If we feel improperly compelled to decide on opposing alternatives, this may mean that we have confused the singular nature of the *res cogitans* with the multiplicity of *res extensa*. Or, we have confused the distinction between soul and body, and this is why the thinker appears to argue for the distinction, for the indivisibility of the soul, so forcefully.

The demon is exorcised only after the soul recognizes its true nature. In essence, the soul is singular, but if it has not learned to control its allocation of free will, it may *feel* as if it is divided, even though this may not really be true. In such an unfortunate confusion of soul and body, little bits of soul can be imagined to have wandered off, and become lost in a substance that is inherently prone to divisibility. The mind feels split up, isolated, disconnected from itself, and with its fragments unable to affect one another. Thus, in certain difficult situations, perhaps only once in a lifetime, those little bits of soul must be gathered up, re-collected, not dismembered, but *re*-membered. In other words, Descartes' hyperbolic doubt may have the specific goal of a *consolidation of consciousness*. This critical moment must precede any subsequent work. It is therefore no wonder the work is called *Meditations on First Philosophy*.

The one small part

Once the soul has gained an understanding of itself, it can then proceed to investigate more deeply the manner in which it is substantially united with the body. The 6th Meditation deals principally with this topic. In the course of this investigation, Descartes (1984) dedicates one small paragraph to a certain location in the body, where it is reasoned to hold an organ of singular importance. This is what would be identified in other works as the pineal gland, or "*conarion*." But in the *Meditations*, he only refers to it, rather coyly, as the "one small part of the brain." This is the one place where all of the different senses come together (p. 59). Notably, this paragraph immediately follows the soul's "indivisibility" argument, mentioned above. However, this description of the pineal gland is noticeably lacking in further detail, which is curious, given how much importance Descartes assigned to it. It is also interesting considering how much this particular assignment has remained with us, in cultural memory. For one example, some have argued that this was the critical step toward a limiting, materialistic view, and Hillman felt that this was the moment in which the soul was banished to imprisonment, for the entirety of the modern era.

Naturally, there is a great deal of misunderstanding on this point as well. In response to Hillman's view, Descartes did not consider the soul to be limited to the pineal gland, only that it holds special importance for the soul's activity. However, both claims are suspect once it is recognized how unique Descartes' reasoning is on this. Essentially, it resonates well with the psychological process currently proposed, and less so than those other accounts might allow.

Along these lines, it is worth noting that Descartes made several observations regarding the pineal gland that were unusually incompatible with the prevailing knowledge of anatomy of his time. Lokhorst (2016) notes that Descartes thought that it occupied a central position, but earlier, Galen had more correctly observed that it did not. Similarly, Descartes believed it to be filled with a very fine wind, but Massa had already observed that it was filled with fluid (para. 14). Lastly, Descartes reasoned that it was very small, and easily movable (para. 20), such that it could be pushed back and forth by the etheric winds of the body, like a ship's sails (para. 14). Not surprisingly, this view of the pineal gland was not well received at the time and was almost universally rejected after his death (para. 40). Therefore, notions much closer to a modern materialistic view can be found both before and after Descartes.

By contrast, Descartes' pineal gland is utterly strange, but makes more sense when compared to his notions of the soul, which have already been established. The soul is, or perhaps must be, indivisible, and also participates primarily in the exercise of free will. For these reasons, the thinker looks for a place in the body that is singular, small, and easily moveable. The body and all its organs, including the heart and the brain, are all divided in two, and thus are not appropriate. The thinker in this case bears some resemblance to the Gnostic myth, that which inventoried all the parts of the body as being in unfortunate pairs. For Descartes, the pituitary gland is singular, but it is observed to be immobile. Descartes only finds the pineal gland to meet all the essential, required conditions.

This is fully articulated from sections of other works. In particular, Descartes' (1985) emphasis on the supposed centrality of the gland is striking. Essentially, the pineal gland is, and must be, in the middle of everything, occupying the "innermost part of the brain." It is in the middle of the senses, the middle of the brain, both left and right halves, as well as front and back (p. 340). As Descartes (1991) describes sensory perception, its central position helps to interpret the dual paths of information. This is because we have two eyes and two ears, and so each side sends a separate stream of information. Again, it is "in the middle of all the concavities" (p. 143). It also occupies a middle position with regard to functionality, having a common mode of operation, which is always the same. This is the case regardless of whether or not the soul acts through it, or if we feel passions, or during sensory perception (Lokhorst, 2016, para. 18).

Although the gland is, in essence, free to move, Descartes (1991) suggests that it may not always be in this state. Some minds are more sluggish than others, perhaps due to excessive memory impressions stored within the pineal gland. By contrast, in the case of "very good and subtle minds, I think the gland must be free from outside influence and easy to move" (p. 143). This formulation accords well with the overall problem of the *Meditations*, in which the mind must be able to free itself from all preconceived opinions. Further, as a result of the prolonged exercise of doubt, the soul eventually discovers its own intrinsic faculties of judgment, and therefore free will. In short, preconceived opinions can weigh down the soul and imprison it, perhaps more so than the body can.

Before leaving the pineal gland, it is worth noting other ways in which it is currently regarded today. The notions of it being a scientific basis for the soul are of course completely extinct. But the pineal gland is thriving in other areas, most notably in Western esotericism, in a way uncannily similar to Descartes' usage. Lokhorst (2016) traces this modern usage back to Madame Blavatsky, who identified the pineal gland as the third eye of the Hindu mystics, an organ of spiritual vision, and this view is immensely popular today (para. 43). In this view, as with Descartes, the gland is not always functional. For Blavatsky, it is currently atrophied (para. 43), but presumably can be re-activated through the practices of, fittingly, *meditation*.

A brief internet search can show that this sentiment is very much alive today. There are innumerable resources that provide specific instructions, including various meditations and other means, on how to "de-calcify" your pineal gland. This would then open the third eye, enabling spiritual visions. "Calcification" naturally invites the suspicion that the gland has become weighed down, and therefore must be cleansed, before it is free to move again. What is most striking about this is that such calcification is not simply from atrophy, but commonly suspected to be the result of malicious governmental influence. It is sometimes suspected that fluoridation of city water is a deliberate attempt to dull our consciousness, reduce our free will, and to keep the public under control. Such means is believed to be developed by the Nazis, but now continues, but only in America (Resnick, 2014).

In these ways, Descartes' concerns may indeed have lived on, although with different terminology and cultural context. Naturally, a direct line of influence from Descartes to these new evaluations is almost unthinkable. This is because Descartes' views were rejected even in his own day, and likely compounded with all the various misunderstandings on his philosophy, even among scholars. However, viewed in terms of an unconscious Anglophone complex, it begins to make some sense.

Recall that complexes manifest in stark polarities of opinion. Fittingly, it seems from this that the pineal gland itself has become split in opinion. There was first the materialistic view, in which Descartes' claims were perhaps not taken seriously enough, and rejected due to lack of empirical backing. Then, there was the spiritual view, led by Blavatsky, who might have taken Descartes' claims too seriously. This divide might have come down through the ages to another, more modern split. Today, Hillman views the gland as a symbol of materialism itself, while the internet practitioners view it as the victim of materialism. That is, it is either the place of the soul's banishment or the exact place through which the soul is trying to express itself.

Overall, it is enough to take all of these modern claims seriously, but more in terms of a symbolic response to split consciousness, rather than literally. This would also extend to Descartes' notions of the pineal gland, especially considering how misplaced it was with the prevailing knowledge of his time, and better placed against a psychological proposition. In other words, it is perhaps best viewed, in all times, as a symbolic image befitting a complex, rather than as any kind of a philosophical or biomedical proposition.

The religious problem

Up until this point, this interpretation of Descartes, particularly of the *Meditations,* is applicable to archetypal split consciousness. That is, even though I have framed it in the context of the Anglophone Cartesian Split complex, it might be relevant to a different cultural complex of a similar nature. This is because archetypes are universal, whereas complexes are always contingent on specific cultures. Therefore, it is conceivable that another culture, with its own traditions and stories, may have formed a different cultural complex, also based on this archetype. This complex would then also have the same characteristics: Atomized units of knowledge and certainty, with no one unit able to be raised above the rest, and with unusual persistence. To this extent, a culture featuring such a complex might be interested in the interpretation offered above. The remainder of this chapter, however, will focus on the Anglophone complex only, the Cartesian Split.

In the previous chapter, I explored how this unique cultural complex carries with it a significant religious concern. Specifically, I suggested that this was related to an unresolved conflict from the English Reformation, which was potentially as unsettling then as it is unrecognized now. This was the pointed rejection of the Medieval practice of the Eucharist, and this created a sort of spiritual void, requiring various substitute images to carry this loss.

In summary, where once there was a meaningful ritual, there were now two conflicting opinions. The Protestant opinion was that the ritual was a fraud, perpetuated by a corrupt priesthood that was only interested in your tithes. Of course, the mass could only be performed by them, to require you to bring those tithes to them. By contrast, the Catholic orthodoxy maintained it as a fact, which you had to accept by faith, however unreasonable it may seem. Thus, faith and reason, tradition and liberation, were split. In between these two increasingly rigid stances, the individual may have been left with some serious doubts on what was really going on, right in front of their eyes.

Again, the *Meditations* deals with a subject of this nature. The thinker entertains similar doubts, by treating all existing opinions, such as those from all the theologians and philosophers, as all equally suspect. One of these sets of opinions is the nature of the body and its relations to the soul. These doubts are internalized, and the thinker plays each off of one another, reaching a high pitch of doubt and confusion, until a solution is found. In the process, the soul is proven to exist, and it is shown that it can find the truth on its own.

However, as dramatic as this is, to encapsulate the whole of the *Meditations* in such a manner risks marginalizing one further aspect of it. Finding truth is one thing, finding truth about the divine is another. However powerful the process of hyperbolic doubt is, and however effective it may resolve a split consciousness, the words and concepts may mean nothing to someone who is struggling with a profound religious crisis.

I believe it would be unwise to underestimate the psychological significance of the loss of such a meaningful religious ritual. Again, this was a ritual that provided physical access to the sacred, providing immediate salvation. And so, the real question may not be so much about how the body is related to the soul, but how the individual is related to God. The crisis of the Reformation indicates that this age-old question may have lost its containment in orthodox ritual, for better or worse. It is fair to surmise that a satisfactory response has yet to be provided. At least, this would seem to be the case, if the only alternatives were to wholly accept the orthodox dogma, or to dogmatically reject it.

Meditations on God

The *Meditations* is many things to many people, but perhaps it is nothing if not considered, first and foremost, as a religious work. Further, it is a cultural product that cannot be wholly extricated from the turmoil of the Reformation. And yet, this is what is normally done. The modern critic of Cartesian dualism usually passes right over the religious problems and focuses only on the philosophical arguments, if he or she even reads the arguments directly. Again, a truly holistic approach would be to look closely at the whole work, and especially the introductory material, where the religious dimensions are immediately apparent. Descartes (1984) dedicates the work to the "sacred Faculty of Theology of Paris," and immediately introduces his reason for writing it. It is not just to introduce a new philosophy, but to also address a religious problem of the day. Further, this is not just the Protestant problem, but that of growing atheism and materialism, which he considers to be the cause of a tragic lack of moral virtue (p. 3). He therefore hopes that the honored Faculty will appreciate his efforts toward maintaining a communal religion. Also, fittingly, its full title is *Meditations on First Philosophy, in which are demonstrated the existence of God and the immortality of the soul.*

It is also fitting that God plays a significant role in the major turning points of the *Meditations*. The first is that of a profound negative presence: The doubt that God even exists. With this move, the thinker takes the arguments of the atheists very seriously. However, this is made worse by suspecting that a malicious demon has filled this void. This was a novel, radical move by Descartes, and it relates to very real fears and anxieties of his peers (Bracken, 2002, pp. 28–31). The first step toward exorcising the demon is to find at least one safe harbor, and this is the *cogito* of the 2nd Meditation.

In the 3rd Meditation, Descartes (1984) deals principally with proving that God exists, and in establishing that God is not a deceiver. What is highly relevant for this study is how the thinker understands his relationship to God. Crucially, there is a distinction between the two, as the thinker is finite and flawed, whereas God is infinite and perfect. However, this does not preclude a relationship in substance, as they are both thinking things (p. 34). Also, this relationship does not consist of a singular event in the past. In the "clockwork" caricature, God made humans as a one-time creation event in the remote past, after which time he is no longer necessary. On the contrary, the thinker realizes himself to be so small and fragile, that he depends on the continual creative influence of God, in order to maintain his existence (p. 33).

The 4th Meditation sets out again to judge truth from deception. However, this is only after the thinker knows he has received the faculty of judgment from a God of truth (Descartes, 1984, p. 37). Also, there is still the problem with how to avoid common human error, which the thinker remembers is all too real. Here is where the role of the will comes in, but again, it is understood in relationship to God. Similar to the nature of ideas, the thinker's will is closely related to God's will, although different in degree (p. 40). The 5th Meditation is a sort of a review, in which God is proved to exist a second time, and as an essential guarantor of knowledge. The 6th Meditation, as stated earlier, focuses on the union of the soul and body, with a short excursion on the pineal gland. Here again, God presides over the body and its various functions, and an understanding is developed of how the soul is to make use of its judgments concerning the body.

Divine substance

With this religious context, a reader having serious doubts on their relationship to God would find some relevant words in this text. In particular, it is interesting to consider closely the substantial relationship between the thinker and God. Both are thinking things, and both are willing things. In the case of the will, the relationship is emphasized even further, as God's will is actually no greater than the thinker's, in "the essential and strict sense" (Descartes, 1984, p. 40). This is even more remarkable considering the perspective of an *Anglophone* reader. English is a peculiar language, and one of its peculiarities is the capitalization of the singular subjective pronoun, the only pronoun that is capitalized. All others, even "me," is not, with the latter not being capitalized because it is the object of some other subject. But when the "I" is the subject, as the prime mover, it is capitalized, as is "God." This is not the case in French and Latin, and so when the text was first translated into English, this relationship was probably unconsciously emphasized.

However, it may still be that the real problem, the loss of meaningful ritual, is left unaddressed. Again, this was a ritual in which Christ's body was reconciled, either re-membered physically, or remembered abstractly. The *Meditations* does not explicitly address this topic, that is, how a mundane substance such as bread relates to a divine substance such as Christ. Correspondingly, it does not concern the question as to who may perform the ritual, or how it was to be done. However, given that these were the hotly debated questions of the day, it is not surprising to see it come up in other works, and this is worth a brief review. Descartes did not publish his *Meditations* alone, but also included a round of critical review from his peers, a set of objections, along with his replies.

In the 4th set of objections, Arnauld (as cited in Descartes, 1984) saves this thorny little problem of the Eucharist for the end. He argues that Descartes' formulation of the substance and accidents of matter does not allow for the miracle of transubstantiation. Thus, he states, "even though [Descartes'] intention was to defend the cause of God against the impious, he may appear to have endangered the very faith" (p. 153). Interestingly this is the Tragic Transcender pattern, but reversed; someone who tried to defend tradition, but unwittingly rejects it.

Descartes (1984) replies to defend his conservative position. First, he contests Arnauld's interpretation of his formulation. Then, he proceeds to argue the opposite, that not only does his formulation allow for the miracle to occur, but that he expects that orthodox theologians will give him a "hearty thanks," for finally providing a clear philosophical basis for a better understanding of the transformation of bread and wine (p. 175). Essentially, he argues that the surfaces of the bread and wine are somewhat distinct from the substance. In other words, that which interacts with our senses is not inherently tied to the underlying change of substance. Thus, Descartes appears to have found, at least for himself, a solution that satisfies the needs of the intellect without threatening the faith.

It is certainly up for debate whether Descartes' offering in this regard is satisfactory. Personally, it seems to me to be a bit strained and defensive, at least from a purely logical perspective. However, what is most interesting to me, and interesting from a standpoint of a psychology of the unconscious, is that he seems to be most careful to preserve an element of mystery.

Mysterious substance

Descartes (1984) does not feel it is necessary to have a detailed explanation of the entire process of transubstantiation. He seems content to account for material substances only to the extent that they activate our senses, leaving the rest open to God's direct influence. He also appeals to common doctrine at the time, that the Real Presence is best understood sacramentally, and perhaps not by reasoning alone. In other words, Christ's body is a "form of existence which we cannot express in words." Rather, our thought depends on being "illumined by faith" (p. 175). Also, earlier, he states, "I firmly insist and believe that many things can be brought about by God which we are incapable of understanding" (p. 173).

With these appeals to preserving mystery, it is certainly fair for a modern critic, looking with modern eyes, to suppose that Descartes is skirting the problem. A similar set of behavior can be found when his critics argue against his famed distinction between mind and body. For, it is said, if the mind and body are two different substances, *how* could they possibly interact? For a modern critic, this one question is believed to be a proper move of checkmate. But for this question as well, Descartes appears to be playing a different game.

This question of interaction was raised, among others, by Gassendi, one of Descartes' harshest critics. In general, Descartes (1984) gets annoyed at such arguments, claiming that they are raised out of ignorance, and so he ignores them (p. 275). Elsewhere, Descartes (1991) states that it is impossible for the human mind to think of the distinction, and their union, at the same time. Even more striking in this reply is that he recommends abstaining from meditation on this point, and to rely primarily on the senses, in order to understand the mind-body union (p. 227). A curious statement from a legendary meditator, and a supposed rationalist!

Critics have often focused on this reply as a betrayal of the fact that his dualism had an unsolvable flaw, and his annoyance and avoidance indicate that, deep down, he probably knew it. Perhaps this is true. However, Descartes (1984) does conclude his reply to Gassendi with one interesting argument that is worth considering. He argues that the conviction that two different substances cannot possibly interact is just another preconceived opinion, which is usually just accepted, but cannot itself be proven (p. 275). Thus, the common argument starts from a foundation that may not be able to survive the process of hyperbolic doubt, if it is carried out properly. Overall, Descartes, for better or worse, is consistent in holding out for a somewhat nonrational conception of substantial interaction.

Again, many volumes have been written on how unsatisfactory this is. As a comprehensive philosophy to explain everything, something Descartes did at times appear to aim for, there are undoubtedly some gaps. The real distinction between mind and body does apparently raise some questions that frustrate the intellect. The long list of Heroic Transcenders, those great thinkers who have all lined up to refute Descartes for the past 350 years, is a powerful testament to this.

However, rather than view this frustration as a flaw in the original idea, something to be refuted, it may in fact be an integral part of the overall psychological situation I am studying. If the *Meditations* can be read as an enactment of a psychological process, addressing the condition of split consciousness, then the presence of frustration may actually be a positive development. That is, it could be a meaningful signal, that the intended resolution to the real problem *is in process*, but perhaps has only been partially reached.

Again, the whole work has to be considered at once, and this would therefore have to fully account for the religious dimension. Regardless of one's religious orientation, a modern reader must admit that the mysterious thinker has undergone some kind of a profound spiritual crisis. Like Dr. Faustus, the thinker may have even gone mad, perhaps even become terrified, and has clearly lost the protection of tradition and the church. He rejects what he once learned of God, and promptly wrestles with an all-powerful demon. He is then dismembered in thought. Only instead of being dragged to hell for eternity, as Faustus was, the thinker has an overwhelming experience of God. Further, it is a God that finally provides an unshakeable truth, a singular truth, and this God remains present, continually preserving all of existence. It is only from this experience that a true understanding is found.

When expressed in such dramatic fashion, it may be more understandable that such an experience allows the thinker to better address the remaining philosophical difficulties. That is, the thinker will now have the ability to know when to stop meditating, and when to allow for the mysteries of what cannot be fully known by the intellect. This may very well be the transformation of substances, or the union of soul and body. And again, such an understanding may be facilitated after having already had a transcendental experience of a good and trustworthy God.

Therefore, *the thinker* may indeed have found a solution to the problem of the Cartesian Split complex, or in other words, how to consolidate a fragmented consciousness, to become whole again. Beyond this, it may also address the Anglophone expression of this problem, the unresolved religious problem of the English Reformation. This was argued to be the loss of a very meaningful ritual, that of the Eucharist, by which mundane substance and divine substance were related. The thinker seems to have found a replacement for this, as he is able to proceed directly from the experience of God, toward having full certainty of the soul's relationship to the body.

However, it is easy to propose that the common reader today may not be able to fully appreciate this or even properly recognize it. From a historical perspective, Descartes' proposed solution was likely ineffective, as the controversies of the Reformation, and those related to them in philosophy, clearly persisted. Such a solution may have even less merit for us today, because in such secular times, we have so few equivalent frames of reference for the original religious problem. On the other hand, there is one frame of reference known today that may offer a new perspective on this very old problem.

Altered substance

Earlier I argued that the *Meditations* may be approached as an enactment of a psychological process, rather than a logical argument. In other words, that the images of hyperbolic doubt, of demons and gods, perhaps even of tragic dismemberment, seem uniquely effective in creating a certain state of mind, from which the remaining work can then proceed. I even suggested that perhaps "no sane person" could properly reach this state of mind. It is therefore possible, and perhaps even likely, that a religious problem such as this requires a "religious" solution. By this, I am suggesting something wholly nonrational.

In other words, the *Meditations* may not only be a work of philosophy or even an early attempt at a psychology. Rather, it could be both of these things, but also taken as a third thing as well. Such a third thing could be disguised in early modern language, but still relevant today. It could be a unique historical record of *an altered state of consciousness.*

There are many good reasons to suppose that the author of the *Meditations* experienced such a state. As the legend goes, Descartes was meditating alone in a stove-heated room, when his thoughts reached such a feverish intensity that he was suddenly and overwhelmingly illuminated with the vision of the "marvelous philosophy." That night, he had his famous three dreams, and these were so meaningful to him, that he vowed the next morning to undertake a spiritual pilgrimage. It is clear from the various sources that this experience was formative to the topics of the *Meditations.* However, a full awareness of this is still relatively young, as early admirers and biographers were unsure how to square such an experience with someone whom they regarded as a master of clear rationalism (Cole, 1992, pp. 6–11; Jones, 1980, p. 145).

What is also relatively young is an academic awareness of the positive benefits of altered, or nonordinary, states of consciousness. There seems to have been a widespread flourishing of this in the mid-20th century, with Aldous Huxley's *Doors of Perception*, and also with the psychedelic research of Timothy Leary, Richard Alpert, and R. Gordon Wasson. Also, much of this work benefitted from contact with indigenous cultures still living in North America, who routinely used psychoactive drugs in ritual. Although initial research was focused heavily on psychedelic *substances*, it has since been well-documented that similar experiences can be produced without such material aid. Psychoactive texts can be just as powerful as psychoactive substances.

In the academic context, altered states of consciousness can be understood to be uniquely therapeutic. They tend to relativize the ego and put it into context with the larger dimensions of the psyche. It is commonly believed that this is equivalent to what prior cultures have called an experience of God (Grof, 2000; Sayin, 2014). The experience is uniquely powerful, to such an extent that new directions in life can be found, where old directions have proven to be limiting. They can also provide meaning, and sometimes are associated with an uncanny increase in knowledge. At the same time, it is also common that a sense of mystery is restored, an understanding that some things cannot be expressed in words. In other words, they are consistent with all of the problems that have been so dutifully raised in the process of the *Meditations*.

A full review of the study of altered states, and their true nature, is far beyond the scope of this work. However, it is very reasonable to assume that before the late 20th century, very few people in the history of Western academia would have known how to properly account for such experiences. In my view, this would certainly include the author of the *Meditations*.

Therefore, it is probable that the author had such an experience, and knew it was enormously valuable, but may have been limited to just that knowledge. He was likely ill-equipped to properly understand it himself, or how to communicate it to others. For this, he can surely be forgiven, as there were no such resources available to him during his time. This may also be why the language may be frustratingly incomplete in this regard, and why the text generated so much controversy.

One thing that we now know of altered states is that they are unique to the individual. No two experiences are ever the same, even to the same person at different times. Thus, the author may have erred in assuming that if he were to simply document the original experience, others would be able to follow along in exactly the same way. Not surprisingly, it may have had the opposite effect on most people, who were perhaps unwilling to enter into an altered state or, in Descartes' words, "meditate seriously with me." This would be for very good reasons, historically. However, even if they were able and willing, the particular constitution of their own individual psychology would likely have required a different kind of experience, in order to accomplish the equivalent goal.

This is not to say that the text was entirely ineffective. It is well known that Leibniz and Spinoza were particularly fascinated with them. Leibniz even went to the trouble of procuring Descartes' private notebook for his own use. Also, both of these great thinkers could certainly be said to have gained an uncanny increase in knowledge, along with a sense of religious mystery, each in his own way.

For the rest of us, however, the text has been preserved merely in the form of a frustration, or as a legendary philosopher who requires continual refutation. On the other hand, again, it could be imagined that the Cartesian Split complex has generated and maintained this frustration for a certain purpose. It may have remained in our cultural memory, as all complexes do, and is activated whenever this particular text is read, as if it knew that it contained within it something important to say. Up until now, this memory may have only manifested in a negative manner, as if saying, this problem will grate on your collective skin, and remain the legendary Cartesian "mind-body problem," until such time as it is newly understood.

Altered meditations

And yet, a final problem remains. If the text can be now understood as an inducer of an altered state of consciousness, addressing the problem of split consciousness, but also insufficient by itself, what else does it require? I am not necessarily advocating here the use of psychedelics, rhythmic movement, trance music, or any other particular method that has been known to facilitate the proper state of mind. However, in the course of this work, I may have provided something equivalent: A new literary context. Particularly, a depth psychological context, with which to frame an old text for a new reading. The entire work that you now hold has thus far been an attempt to establish an archetypal, mythic framework for the tragedy of the Cartesian Split. I intentionally selected and transcribed the most powerful and moving rhetoric from all the critiques, preserving the most detailed psychological images. For this reason, it is no longer necessary to refer to these critiques as products of a cultural complex. Rather, I see them all as helpful constructs of a new myth. Perhaps it is these mythic words that can generate the necessary state of mind, simply from reading them thoroughly, or meditating on them seriously. If so, the problem of split consciousness could finally be read in its proper, native language.

This is the language of the archetype of Dismemberment, which has a definite lineage, going back all the way to antiquity. Empedocles recognized that the separation of elements was a fundamental process, inherent to the very fabric of creation, but that also the process of reconciliation can go very wrong, with sometimes horrifying results. Similarly, all of the creation myths referenced thus far featured at least a dark overtone, regarding this original separation. This tone was progressively emphasized, with Zeus viciously splitting humans apart, and then to the Gnostic demiurge, who presided over a perpetual split between Heaven and Earth, between Mind and Body. Then, there was the tragedy of Dr. Faustus, who dared to internalize such splitting, and work out his own solution to this age-old conflict. The poor doctor ended up violently dismembered, and scattered on dung heaps. But where Faustus failed, the Thinker now appears, and has claimed to have worked out a solution. All of these stories, when taken together, and culminating in the re-reading of the *Meditations* as a potential answer, may provide for the necessary foundation, for a much-needed new style of consciousness, today.

These are all archetypal stories, and archetypes are activated when reading them. They are the deep structures of the psyche, the images of our instincts. As such, when something goes wrong with the psyche, they have the ability to get things back on the right path. They can also provide for an increased understanding, a sense of meaning, and set out new directions for life. And overall, they can create an experience of the numinous and a restoration of mystery. Jung believed that the culminating experience of individuation was the ego's experience of the Self, and that this was also an experience of God. To the extent that the Thinker's God does not hold meaning for us, it is then up to us, to develop the rest on our own.

References

Baker, G. P., & Morris, K. J. (2002). *Descartes' dualism*. London, UK: Routledge.

Bordo, S. (1987). *The flight to objectivity: Essays on Cartesianism and culture*. Albany: State University of New York Press.

Bracken, H. M. (2002). *Descartes*. Oxford, UK: Oneworld.

Cole, J. R. (1992). *The Olympian dreams and youthful rebellion of René Descartes*. Urbana: University of Illinois Press.

Descartes, R. (1984). *The philosophical writings of Descartes* (Vol. 2; J. Cottingham, R. Stoothoff, & D. Murdoch, Trans.). Cambridge, UK: Cambridge University Press.

Descartes, R. (1985). *The philosophical writings of Descartes* (Vol. 1; J. Cottingham, R. Stoothoff, & D. Murdoch, Trans.). Cambridge, UK: Cambridge University Press.

Descartes, R. (1991). *The philosophical writings of Descartes* (Vol. 3; J. Cottingham, R. Stoothoff, D. Murdoch, & A. Kenny, Trans.). Cambridge, UK: Cambridge University Press.

Eshleman, M. (2007). The Cartesian unconscious. *History of Philosophy Quarterly*, *24*(2), 169–187.

Frankfurt, H. G. (2008). *Demons, dreamers, and madmen: The defense of reason in Descartes's meditations*. Princeton, NJ: Princeton University Press.

Grof, S. (2000). *Psychology of the future: Lessons from modern consciousness research*. Albany: State University of New York Press.

Hutton, S. (2013). The Cambridge platonists. In E. N. Zalta (Ed.), *The Stanford encyclopedia of philosophy*. Retrieved from: https://plato.stanford.edu/archives/win2013/entries/cambridge-platonists/

Jones, W. T. (1980). Somnio ergo sum: Descartes's three dreams. *Philosophy and Literature*, *4*(2), 145–162.

Jung, C. G. (1969a). A review of the complex theory. In R. F. C. Hull (Trans.), *The collected works of C. G. Jung* (Vol. 8, pp. 92–104). Princeton, NJ: Princeton University Press. (Original work published 1934)

Jung, C. G. (1969b). Conscious, unconscious, and individuation. In R. F. C. Hull (Trans.), *The collected works of C. G. Jung* (Vol. 9.1, pp. 275–289). Princeton, NJ: Princeton University Press. (Original work published 1954)

Jung, C. G. (1970). A psychological view of conscience. In R. F. C. Hull (Trans.), *The collected works of C. G. Jung* (Vol. 10, pp. 437–455). Princeton, NJ: Princeton University Press. (Original work published 1958)

Kelso, C. (2015, February 10). Reuniting the apparent mind/body split. Retrieved February 17, 2019, from The Deepest Peace website: https://thedeepestpeace.com/2015/02/10/reuniting-the-apparent-mindbody-split/#more-413

Lee, K. (2013). *Reading Descartes otherwise: Blind, mad, dreamy, and bad*. New York, NY: Fordham University Press.

Lokhorst, G. (2016). Descartes and the pineal gland. In E. N. Zalta (Ed.), *The Stanford encyclopedia of philosophy*. Retrieved from: http://plato.stanford.edu/archives/sum2016/entries/pineal-gland/

Morris, K. (in press). The real distinction between mind and body. Forthcoming. In C. Lim & J. Secada (Eds.), *The Cartesian mind*. London, UK: Routledge.

https://www.amazon.co.uk/Cartesian-Mind-Routledge-Philosophical-Minds/dp/1138847429

Morris, K. (2017). The hard problem of understanding Descartes on consciousness. In D. Jaquette (Ed.), *The Bloomsbury companion to the philosophy of consciousness* (pp. 11–26). London, UK: Bloomsbury.

Resnick, J. (2014, April 25). The effects of fluoride on consciousness and the will to act. Retrieved April 2, 2017, from The Conscious Reporter website: http://consciousreporter.com/conspiracy-against-consciousness/the-effects-of-fluoride-on-consciousness-and-the-will-to-act/

Sayin, H. Ü. (2014). Does the nervous system have an intrinsic archaic language? Entoptic images and phosphenes. *NeuroQuantology*, *12*(3), 427–445. doi: 10.14704/nq.2014.12.3.756

Index

Made in the USA
Las Vegas, NV
19 September 2026

8f314054-1812-45e3-a46f-e991ada320d5R01